Best Care Anywhere

Best Care Anywhere

Why VA Health Care Is Better Than Yours

SECOND EDITION

PHILLIP LONGMAN

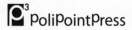

Best Care Anywhere:
Why VA Health Care Is Better Than Yours,
Second Edition

© 2010 by Phillip Longman

14   13   12   11   10   2   3   4   5

Production management: BookMatters
Book design: BookMatters
Cover design: Nicole Hayward

Library of Congress Cataloging-in-Publication Data
    Longman, Phillip.
        Best care anywhere : why VA health care is better
    than yours / Phillip Longman. — 2nd ed.
            p. ; cm.
        Includes bibliographical references and index.
        ISBN 978-0-9824171-5-7 (alk. paper)
        1. United States. Dept. of Veterans Affairs.
    2. Veterans—Medical care—United States.
    3. Medical care—United States. I. Title.
    [DNLM: 1. United States. Veterans Administration.
    2. Delivery of Health Care—United States.
    3. Hospitals, Veterans—United States.   4. Quality
    of Health Care—United States. W 84 AA1 L856b
    2010]
    UB369.L66   2010
    362.1086'970973—dc22   2010004038

Published by:
PoliPointPress, LLC
80 Liberty Ship Way, Suite 22
Sausalito, CA 94965
(415) 339-4100
www.polipoint.com

Distributed by Ingram Publisher Services

Printed in the USA

Contents

Preface to the Second Edition

A month after *Best Care Anywhere* first appeared in January 2007, the *Washington Post* began an exposé on problems at Walter Reed Army Medical Center in Washington, DC—a series for which it later won the Pulitzer Prize. The facility is a U.S. Army hospital, as its name indicates, run by the Department of Defense, not by the separate cabinet agency— the Department of Veterans Affairs (VA)—whose virtues I had described in my book. Nonetheless, this distinction was lost in much of the reporting on the scandal, leaving many Americans with the impression that the VA was neglecting grievously wounded warriors. As media and congressional investigations mounted, my publisher and editor pretty well gave up on the book, as they later told me. Meanwhile, I endured blogosphere ridicule for having written one of the worst-timed books in years.

Yet slowly, by word of mouth, the book and its paradoxical message began to attract positive notice and to exert some influence behind the scenes. For example, in an odd loop the loop, when reporters around the country started visiting their local VA hospitals looking for scandalous conditions like those described by the *Post* at Walter Reed, they often came away as impressed as I had been in researching my book. The VA received an unexpected burst of positive coverage, in which *Best Care Anywhere* was often cited. That coverage has continued to build; the *Wall Street Journal* is the latest organ of the mainstream media to discover the virtues of the VA's model of care.[1]

Behind the scenes, people in high places, as well, became aware of the quality revolution at the VA that I had described. For example, in the spring of 2007, I was twice summoned to brief the health-care staff of then leading Democratic presidential candidate Hillary Clinton. Afterward, her standard speech on health-care quality came to include two paragraphs on the transformation of the nation's long-tarnished veterans' health-care system and its lessons for improving quality in health care generally.

Through a well-placed friend and colleague, a copy of the book was also slipped to candidate Barack Obama before he boarded a long flight to Hawaii. Whether he read it, I do not know, but he, too, began making positive references to the VA in his health-care addresses. Peter Orszag, then director of the Congressional Budget Office and now Obama's head of the Office of Management and Budget, began ordering up studies from his staff on the lessons of the VA's quality performance.[2]

Interest stirred in some Republican circles as well. Michael Cannon, director of health policy studies at the libertarian Cato Institute, took exception to the idea that the VA—the nation's one undeniable example of fully socialized medicine—should stand as a model of twenty-first-century health reform. But he acknowledged the VA's emergence as a quality leader in health care and wrote thoughtfully for the *National Review* about how the agency's performance might be replicated in the private sector.[3]

Already resigned to the seemingly irresistible trend toward more government spending on health care, at least a few "Blue Dog" Democrats began quietly consulting with me about whether the VA's proven efficiency might offer clues for containing health-care costs generally. Speaking invitations at Yale, the University of Pennsylvania (Wharton School of Business), and other universities, as well as increasing sales to university bookstores, also signaled increasing academic interest. Through the initiative of academics in Beijing University, the book is also being translated into Chinese. (As the U.S.'s prime creditor, China is particularly interested these days to learn if a model exists, such as a civilian version of the VA, for containing the spiraling cost of the U.S. health-care system, because otherwise, China worries, we won't be able to repay our mounting debts.)

Interest in the book also began to spread among the larger veterans' community. Organizations such as the American Legion are often heard in the media and in Congress complaining about the VA's shortfalls, as is their role. They are particularly upset, and rightly so, about how difficult it can be for veterans to establish eligibility for VA care. But they are also tenacious in their advocacy for the VA and its ongoing quality revolution in ways that offer fascinating soundings into the deeper currents of American health-care politics. During the summer of 2009, I had the great honor of addressing a large audience of American Legion officials at their annual convention in Louisville, Kentucky. Looking back at me was an assemblage of many middle-aged and older vets, mostly drawn from small-town, Red-State America. Steeped in patriotic traditions and bedecked with its symbols, they spontaneously stood and cheered when I suggested that they tell their neighbors about today's VA—and about the ability of "socialized medicine" to deliver the "Best Care Anywhere."

Yet it is fair to say that outside of the very different worlds of health-care policy wonks and veteran service organizations, the VA's reputation remains mixed at best. This divided reputation is partly due to the VA's long history, particularly during the Vietnam era, as a deeply troubled institution. That legacy still affects its image. Many Americans simply have not heard of the VA's quality transformation, and even when they have, they remain skeptical because of their generally dim view of government.

The VA's mixed reputation is also partly due to the fact that its mistakes tend to become national news. The recent headlines include surgical malfeasance associated with the deaths of nine veterans at the VA's facility in Marion, Illinois. In Philadelphia, a rogue surgeon, employed by the University of Pennsylvania but under contract with the VA, improperly treated prostate cancer patients with a life-threatening nuclear procedure. These examples of malpractice are egregious, but in gauging their significance, we must ask, "Compared to what?" Medical errors are demonstrably less common in the VA than elsewhere in the health-care sector, and study after study demonstrates the VA's superior quality of care. But because of the public nature of the VA, and because the VA systematically looks for and reports its mistakes, those errors are much more likely to come to public attention, through congressional hearings, press reports, and investigations by veterans advocacy groups and the VA's own inspector general. The cumulative effect on the average news consumer can be an impression that the VA is limping along from one scandal to the next, even as its patients and health-care quality experts applaud its quality, safety, and cost-effectiveness.

Until recently, this gap in the public's understanding of the VA's story didn't much figure in practical, day-to-day politics. That's because the country's political system was caught up in a protracted debate that largely ignored reform of the actual practice of medicine. Almost all the arguments about health care in recent years have really been about heath care *insurance*—who should get it, and who should pay for it. Little thought has been given to reform of the health-care delivery system. This focus on insurance has left the VA's story, which is about a proven model of safe, efficient, digitally driven, evidence-based medicine, largely out of the conversation except in specialized health-care policy circles.

When *Best Care Anywhere* was first published, for example, a Republican White House was arguing that unsustainable health-care inflation could only be checked if Americans came to "have more skin in the game," that is, to pay more of the cost of their health care out of their own pockets. Measures such as health savings accounts and high-deductible insurance plans were supposed to encourage patients to do more comparison shopping and haggling with their doctors and therefore to create more market discipline in the system. Essentially, this remains the Republican position on health care.

Meanwhile, the dominant idea for health-care reform among centrist Democrats was and remains the "individual mandate," as championed by presidential candidate Hillary Clinton and later by President Obama and the Democratic Party leadership in Congress. The proposal, one version of which passed the House and Senate as of this writing (but which is also rapidly losing popular support), would require all Americans to purchase health insurance; those who cannot afford the premiums would get subsidies. This arrangement would, by fiat, end or at least reduce the problem of the uninsured and also promises to prevent private insurance companies from discriminating against people suffering from preexisting conditions.

Further to the Left are people who have argued, and still argue, that health-care reform simply entails creation of a "single-payer system," specifically a policy that would extend Medicare-like insurance coverage to everyone. Short of that policy, the progressive cry has been for a "public option" that would give at least some Americans the opportunity to purchase government-provided health *insurance*, though not government-provided health *care*.

Given this spectrum of opinion, the VA model's advantages in the hands-on delivery of health care have hardly been part of the national debate. Many insiders say that this low profile is necessary. Political logic dictates, they have argued, that first we insure the uninsured, and later we worry about what we have insured them against—that is, what protocols of health care Americans should receive for different conditions and how to ensure their delivery. Less charitably, future historians may look back at the terms of our recent health-care debate and view them as part of a larger, darker cultural phenomenon of our time.

An odd feature of the last few decades of American life has been the tendency, especially among the "best and brightest," to focus not on hands-on production, whether it be of automobiles, homes, or health care, but on "derivatives" of production—the manipulation of symbols that has become the essence of finance, from securitized auto loans and subprime mortgages to high-deductible or public option health insurance policies. Yet now we are reaching a moment when continuing the conflation of finance with production—and particularly of health-care finance with health care itself—has played out about as far as it usefully can.

To be sure, health insurance reform is important. Done right, it can remove some of the most egregious conditions of American life: the discrimination against the sick in insurance markets, such as my late wife, Robin, and I faced during her losing battle with breast cancer; the uniquely American phenomenon of medical bankruptcy; the tens of thousands of premature deaths among the un- and under-insured; and wasteful flows of funds going to maximize insurance company profits and to bloat administrative costs. Through adjustments in fee schedules and in the terms of reimbursement contracts with doctors and hospitals, insurance could also, at least in theory, indirectly influence medical practice for the better. But make no mistake: none of the health insurance reforms we've been so strongly debating will, by themselves, solve the health-care crisis, and expanding access to an already broken, fragmented, and overwhelmed health-care delivery "system" could well make it worse.

In updating the statistics for this edition, I have been reminded again and again of the continuing breakdown of day-to-day medical practice in the United States: the extraordinary levels of unnecessary and often harmful treatments; the high rates of medical errors and of untreatable hospital infections; the neglect of prevention, of primary care, of patient safety, of coordination among specialists, of basic research on what works and doesn't, of investment in simple health information technology for purposes beyond billing.

It all brings to mind a concept that encapsulates all these and other baleful trends in our health-care delivery system: iatrogenesis. The term, coined by the ancient Greeks, refers to death and suffering caused by poor medical treatment or advice. Today, iatrogenesis includes unnecessary surgery, medical errors, hospital-acquired infections, and the prescribing of unsafe drugs or unsafe combinations of drugs. According to an estimate published in the *Journal of the American Medical Association*, such iatrogenic practices minimally kill 225,000 Americans per year. This rate makes contact with the American health system the third-largest cause of death in the United States, following heart disease and all cancers.[4]

By contrast, a widely accepted 2002 estimate by the Institute of Medicine holds that 18,000 Americans die every year because of lack of health insurance. Though some believe this estimate is too low, even the direst projections would mean that iatrogenic medicine (most of it covered by insurance) kills five times more Americans.[5]

Moreover, a fair accounting of iatrogenic medicine must also include the less quantifiable but nonetheless undeniable illness and suffering induced by wasteful spending on health care itself, whether that spending is borne by individuals or society as a whole. Numerous studies now confirm that about a third of all health-care spending is pure waste, mostly in the form of unnecessary and often harmful care—amounting to some $700 billion a year.[6] That's $56 billion more than total federal spending in 2009 for Social Security, a program that, along with many other programs, may well have to be cut to cover the soaring cost of Medicare and Medicaid. Already, a nation spending that much on wasteful health care is a nation that necessarily spends less than it otherwise could on reducing the major social and economic determinants of illness, including unemployment, lack of education, pollution, addiction, poor nutrition, auto dependency, and strains between work and family life. Whether today's U.S. healthcare system is, on balance, iatrogenic—that is, contributing, directly and indirectly, to more illness than it cures—cannot be conclusively demonstrated. But it is at least a possibility, and one that becomes increasingly certain given current trends.

So the moment comes when we must move beyond the realm of mere finance and be as empirical as we can about what works and does not work in the delivery of health care. The central contention of the current administration's vision for putting America back on course, let us not forget, is that our health-care system today is so wasteful and poorly organized that we can lower costs, expand access, and raise quality all at the same time—and even have money left over at the end to help pay for other major programs, from bank bailouts to high-speed rail. It is not too much to say that the Obama administration is betting the country on this proposition, or would like to.

The proposition is not as implausible at it might sound. America spends nearly twice as much per person as other developed countries for health outcomes that are no better. The cost of health care has become so gigantic that pushing down its growth rate by just 1.5 percentage points per year would free up more than $2 trillion over the next decade, which would buy a lot of high-speed trains and much else that our country needs, from investment in green energy and infrastructure repair to the retooling of America's manufacturing base and the employment of its laid-off workers. It could also allow for a nice-sized tax cut, if that turns out to be our preference, or for a large down payment on the ballooning national debt. But bending that health-care cost curve requires fundamentally changing the practice of medicine, not just its financing.

The VA system is hardly a perfect model for a delivery system reform. Yet its comparative effectiveness should be examined and explained if we are to have any hope of building a world-class health-care system that is not itself a major cause of death, suffering, impoverishment, and national decline.

By all rights, after all, the VA should offer the worst care anywhere: it's a gigantic, unionized bureaucracy, micromanaged by Congress and political appointees, and beset by an uncertain budget, an aging infrastructure, and a legacy of scandal. That it nonetheless outperforms the rest of the U.S. health-care system, on metrics ranging from patient satisfaction to cost-effectiveness and the use of evidence-based medicine, suggests that much of what we think we know about health care simply isn't true. The VA's long-term relationship with its patients, it turns out, more than makes up for its built-in institutional liabilities, which offers a lesson for health-care reform that we ignore at our peril. I offer this second edition of *Best Care Anywhere* in the hope that more readers worried about their own health and that of the nation will consider the meaning of the VA's paradoxical example and its implications for true health-care reform.

January 20, 2010,
Washington, DC

Introduction

Some years ago, *Fortune* magazine summoned me to New York for a sumptuous lunch and a serious discussion. At the end of the meal, I found myself with a plum, but difficult, freelance assignment. It was no less than to figure out who had the best solutions for America's health-care crisis, and to write them up in snappy prose that would make the story a "must read" for the country's business elite. What the magazine had in mind, I think, was that I find some dynamic, change-artist CEO who was doing for health care what Andrew Grove had once done for Intel or what Jack Welch had done for General Electric.

I accepted these marching orders with much trepidation, but also great curiosity and passion. The biggest reason was personal. Five years before, I had lost my wife, Robin, to breast cancer. I never blamed her doctors for her death. But what I saw of the American health-care system during the 10 months between her diagnosis and demise had caused me to stop regarding health care as a mere abstraction. I had become personally engaged in the question of how the American health-care system actually worked, or all too often, didn't work.

Robin was treated at the prestigious Lombardi Cancer

Center, part of Georgetown University's hospital, in upscale Northwest Washington, DC. Every time she and I entered the facility through its posh lobby, we passed a poster-sized blowup, mounted on an easel, of a recent cover of *U.S. News & World Report* that ranked Lombardi as one of the best cancer treatment centers in the country. Since I worked at *U.S. News* at the time and respected the team responsible for these annual rankings, this was particularly reassuring.

Robin and I both felt blessed that our gold-plate insurance allowed us unfettered access to all the doctors and specialists we would care to see, and that we lived within just a short drive of Lombardi's world-class facilities. I particularly remember Robin saying how grateful she was that we hadn't chosen to try to save money by enrolling with an HMO. We were lucky yuppies, and we knew it.

Yet the more time we spent in the Lombardi Center and Georgetown Hospital, the more I was disturbed by the way they managed "the little things." On the day Robin underwent her lumpectomy, for example, I had to explain to her afterwards as best I could why I wasn't there to offer her support and comfort when she awoke. The reason, though hard for both of us to believe at the time, was that no one in the hospital could tell me, despite my increasingly frantic inquiries, where she was. I had imagined that every hospital, particularly a prestigious one attached to a major university in the nation's capital, operated with advanced information technology systems that kept track of every patient's location and condition. Not true, it turns out.

I was similarly shocked at how little the various specialists involved in her care seemed to consult with one another, or to keep up to date on the results of tests. In one emotionally devastating meeting, for example, the discussion began with various members of Robin's "team" optimistically discussing her prospects for reconstructive surgery. Robin and I were both thrilled that the lumpectomy was an apparent success and that her chemotherapy seemed to be working to contain the cancer. But well into the meeting, one doctor began to fidget, finally asking if anyone had looked at the results of a recent liver scan. The team quickly departed, leaving Robin and me in an empty examining room for 30 or 40 minutes. Eventually, a grim-faced oncologist returned. The cancer had metastasized to her liver. It looked as if she was terminal.

As I said, I never blamed her doctors for her death, but seeds of doubt sprouted in my mind about the system in which they were operating. Most of the doctors were sympathetic enough, and all were highly credentialed. But there seemed to be little attention given to managing information and coordinating care. It was as if, upon arriving at an airline gate, you were informed that the airline had lost track of the plane, couldn't find its passenger manifest, and couldn't say if it had passed its last inspection. At any given time, Robin's medical records and test results seemed to be scattered in paper files kept by different departments. If any one doctor played the role of pilot, much less air traffic controller, I had no idea who he or she was.

The experience of Robin's treatment set off unsettling questions in my mind, though I tried to suppress them. Who was in charge of quality control? Why did everything seem to be done on the fly? Why did almost every routine process—doctor visits, lab tests, chemotherapy sessions—seem to involve interminable waits or changes in plan? I couldn't offer Robin any comfort either when she received the news that she only had an estimated 17 days to live and would have to go home from the hospital to die. A doctor had changed his mind without telling us about when he would share with us the results of Robin's latest tests. And so she received this death sentence while alone in the hospital and had no one to talk to about it for hours. In a normal business, such as an airline, being perpetually late and having to shift plans constantly are sure signs that its processes are breaking down and that something bad is waiting to happen.

Then there were all the logistical and insurance issues. When was someone going to change her IV? When could our two-year-old son visit her? How long could she stay in the hospital after she had been declared terminal? How could one arrange for home hospice care, what did it cost, and who would pay? I came away feeling that no patient should ever enter a hospital without having some kind of full-time advocate—a caring, calm, and shrewd relative or friend at least, preferably with medical training and a law degree—to help navigate all the potential perils. And I wondered why the American health-care system, or at least this one prestigious corner of it, had come to be like this.

A short time after Robin died, I read in the newspaper that the Institute of Medicine had issued a landmark report in which it estimated that up to 98,000 Americans were killed every year in hospitals as a result of medical errors—a toll which exceeded that of AIDS, breast cancer, or even motor vehicle accidents. The article also put it another way: It was like three jumbo jets crashing every other day and killing all on board. I was shocked, but upon reflection, not incredulous.[1]

Indentured Servitude

Another reason I was eager to accept *Fortune*'s assignment was that the American health-care crisis seemed finally to be coming to a head. As long ago as 1970, the editors of *Fortune* had put out a special issue on medical care, declaring it "on the brink of chaos." *BusinessWeek,* that same year, had a cover story on American health care titled "$60 Billion Crisis." But health care by now was close to a $2 *trillion* crisis, and that didn't even count all the indirect costs it was imposing on the economy and Americans' pursuit of happiness.

One of those indirect costs that I, along with millions of other Americans, had experienced firsthand was finding myself trapped in a job by my need for insurance. Shortly after Robin's cancer was diagnosed, *U.S. News* went through a management shakeup. The editor who had hired me was summarily fired, and I found myself on the losing side of a regime change. The jig was up, and it was time for me to go.

But, though I had several tempting offers, I had to stay and tough it out as best I could because I could not risk changing insurance plans with Robin's preexisting condition. As it turned out, I was fortunate to be able to keep my job for as long as I had to, and I'm very grateful to all involved for that. But the experience sensitized me to how many Americans are stuck in place year after year—unable to start a new business, go back to school, or even take time off to care for a loved one—just because of the way we finance our health-care system.

I was also aware, of course, of the many familiar trend lines that make our health-care system unsustainable. Two years before Robin died, when our son was born prematurely at just 2½ pounds, I was amazed by and grateful to doctors and nurses at Sarasota Memorial Hospital who managed to keep him alive. But during the 60 days he was in the neonatal intensive care ward, I came to know other parents of "pree-mies" who, regardless of whether they lost their babies, were losing their homes and headed toward bankruptcy because they lacked health insurance. Since then, the number of such tragedies has only grown.

Every year, the cost of health care rises faster than the economy grows, with results that are as predictable as they are depressing. Because of its soaring price, we see millions of workers forced to forgo raises and to assume more and more of the cost of their health care, even if they are still lucky enough to have group insurance. We see the crush of medical expenses emerging as the number one source of personal bankruptcy.[2] We see once-proud corporations like General Motors made wards of the state and forced to downsize in large part because of their ruinous liabilities for employee and retiree health-care benefits. We see state and local governments raising taxes and the federal government going deeper and deeper in debt as they try to cover the exploding cost of publicly financed health-care programs. And all this inflation and economic turmoil just as the baby boomers, my generation, begin experiencing the infirmities and chronic illnesses of old age. At current growth rates, health-care spending is projected to consume anywhere from 119 percent to 142 percent of the entire real increase in U.S. per capita income over the next 75 years, sucking trillions of dollars away from other vital purposes.[3] Can health-care spending at that level even begin to ameliorate the ill health it would cause? Such a price would necessarily reduce, as it is reducing today, the amount of time and money left for educating children, fighting poverty, cleaning up the environment, fostering community, and relieving all the other socioeconomic determinants of illness.

Health Care's Declining Pace of Progress

A final reason I was eager to take on *Fortune*'s assignment was a little-known but diabolical fact I had stumbled upon shortly after Robin died. The more I thought about it, the more alarming and outrageous it seemed to me. I discovered it after reading a study by the Federal Reserve that calculated how many hours, in different eras, the average American worker had to be on the job to make enough money to purchase various big-ticket items.

The study showcased the example of cars. Back in 1955, for instance, the average worker had to labor 1,638 hours to earn enough to buy a brand new Ford Fairlane. By 1997, the average American worker earned enough in just 1,365 hours to buy a brand new Ford Taurus, which, unlike the Fairlane, came with such standard features as air conditioning, airbags, cruise control, and power windows, steering, and brakes, and it got much better mileage. According to the study, a similar pattern of improving quality at lower real cost is true of nearly every big-ticket item for sale in the American economy.[4]

But what, I wondered, would happen if one included the cost of health care, which the study did not? It's a simple calculation, and when I did the math, the results were as devastating as they were revealing. If you've ever wondered how the nation's per capita GDP can grow year after year without most Americans feeling any richer, here's a big part of the explanation.

Let's travel back to 1964, for example. Most Americans were feeling prosperous. Suburbia was burgeoning. Record numbers of American youth were becoming the first in their families to go to college. Intellectuals complained about the miseries of "The Affluent Society." Yet the average American worker took home only $2.53 an hour. How does that square? You can't just say that a dollar went further in those days, because as we've just seen, the real cost of cars and just about every other consumer item has actually declined since that era. But there is a ready explanation. While workers in the 1960s had to put in many more hours on the job to purchase items like televisions, cars, or a ride in an airplane, they hardly had to work at all to cover the cost of health care. At the time, health-care spending in the United States was just $197 per person per year. This low cost meant that with a mere 78 hours of labor (or by the end of the second work week in January, for those working full time), the average worker earned enough to cover the per capita cost of health care, including that of all children and retirees.

By contrast, in 2007, despite massive improvements in productivity outside the health-care sector, the average worker had to put in 411 hours before earning enough to cover the average per capita burden of medical expenses, which by then had risen to over $6,300. Put another way, in that year it was well into March before the average American, working a 40-hour week, earned enough to pay the health-care sector's growing claim on personal output.

Given current trends in wages and health-care spending, by 2054, the average American worker will need to devote 2,970 hours a year to cover the cost of health care. That would mean working at least 8 hours a day, every day of the year, from January to December, with all of life's needs outside of health care somehow financed by still more exertion. So much for the Affluent Society. Obviously, something big is going to give.

It gets worse when you think about it. What kind of health care did Americans get back in 1964 for just $197? For those too young to remember that era, health care back then was far from primitive. A strong memory I have from childhood is that of my maternal grandfather explaining to me, sometime in the mid-'60s, how he could not in good conscience continue practicing medicine because it had become too sophisticated, complicated, and fast paced for him to follow any longer. He had graduated from the University of Michigan's medical school in 1927 as part of a new generation of doctors whose training was rigorous, competitive, and grounded in science, and he had gone on to enjoy a distinguished career in medicine. But by the mid-1960s he felt out of his depth.

The operations performed in that era included open-heart surgery, the implanting of pacemakers, and neurosurgery for the treatment of Parkinson's disease and other neurological disorders. Electrocardiograms were in common use, and doctors had long since learned how to use defibrillation to jump-start stalled hearts. My own mother almost died of a misdiagnosed appendicitis in the 1960s, but once the right diagnosis was made, she was easily saved by an appendectomy, which by then had become a routine operation.

Thanks to the increasing use of kidney dialysis machines, death rates from kidney disease were also plunging. Anesthesia no longer just meant knocking patients out with ether; it included local anesthesia, pain management, resuscitation, oxygen therapy, and the use of mechanical ventilators to avoid lung complications in patients recovering from major surgery. The polio vaccine was fully developed, and tuberculosis was nearly vanquished, as were such devastating child killers as diphtheria and whooping cough. Wonder drugs like penicillin and other new antibiotics had caused the death rate from pneumonia and other infectious diseases to plummet.

In all the time I spent growing up in the 1960s, I knew only one classmate who died from a childhood disease, and I knew none who lost a parent to illness. Then, as now, cancer patients were treated with prolonged chemotherapy, the development of which had been generously supported by government funding since the mid-1950s. Doctors did not yet have PET scans or MRIs, but X-rays achieved much the same purpose and in any event required expensive equipment and highly trained personnel.

The quality of doctors was also very high. Long gone were the quacks who had typified American medicine at the beginning of the century. By the 1960s, even elderly doctors, such as my maternal grandfather, had undergone medical training as prolonged and exacting as that received by doctors today, including a minimum of 4 years of medical school and at least 1 year of postgraduate internship. Though most physicians may not have lived up to the performance of such celebrated television doctors of the era as Marcus Welby, MD, and Dr. Kildare, polling data clearly show that health-care leaders in that era enjoyed a reputation for probity and professionalism that is long gone today.[5]

Hospitals in the 1960s also offered levels of service as high as, and in some ways higher than, they typically do now. Private and semiprivate rooms were already the norm. In the 1960s, patients were also allowed to stay in the hospital much longer than today, which of course cost money. Not all of those extra days were medically necessary, but it would have been considered malpractice to send home patients who still required infusions or highly flammable oxygen tanks, as is routinely done today. Nor would hospitals simply send terminally ill patients home to die with a stash of morphine and some counseling from a social worker, which, as I discovered with Robin, is too often the present-day meaning of home "hospice" care.

A Mexican acquaintance, who used to work in a store near our house, couldn't believe it when I told him, shortly after Robin died, the reason he hadn't seen me in 2 weeks. I explained that, with no hospice beds available at nearby institutions, I'd been holed up with my mother at home, with barely time to eat or sleep, trying to tend to Robin in her final days while at the same time looking after a very upset and angry two-year-old who couldn't bear to watch his mother slowly die before his eyes. "In Mexico," the man said, shaking his head, "we never send people home to die."

Hospitals in the 1960s also routinely bore the cost of providing a calm, safe place for alcoholics to detox and for the emotionally distraught to have their "nervous breakdowns"— services that are today usually offered on an "outpatient" basis. Again, providing these services in the hospital was not always the most cost-effective option, but these services were part of what Americans got from the health-care system for just $197 per year, or just 2 weeks' labor.

So why does the average American now have to work until mid-March of every year to earn the per capita cost of health care? Where is all this money going? And what improvements in health is it buying? Here the facts get even more outrageous. Yes, many individuals today owe their lives to treatments that were unavailable a generation ago. These notably include timely treatments in emergency rooms, which were still uncommon in the 1960s. (Though these days, emergency room treatments are maybe not so timely—if you arrive at the ER on a Friday night, you may wait through the weekend to be treated for a nonlethal condition.) We've also become much better at keeping underweight babies alive. Elective treatments like cataract surgery have improved the quality of many people's lives. And yes, since the passage of Medicare and Medicaid in 1965, the poor and elderly have far better access to health care than they previously did.

But for the population as a whole, the results in improved health and life expectancy are astonishingly modest. The rate of improvement in life expectancy, for example, actually slowed substantially after the explosion in health-care spending that began in the 1960s. Between 1900 and 1960, life expectancy at birth in the United States increased by an average of 0.64 percent per year. From 1960 to 2004, however, that rate of improvement declined by 40 percent, to just 0.24 percent per year.[6] Moreover, the gains in life expectancy that have been achieved over the last 40 years have come largely from broad social and technological trends, not strictly from medical interventions.

For example, today's Americans smoke far less, drive far safer cars, run much less risk of being injured on the job, and are much less likely to be shot accidentally, to cite just four major nonmedical sources of increased longevity. From 1960 to 2002, the age-adjusted death rate from unintentional injuries, such as from car wrecks, firearm accidents, and on-the-job accidents, declined by 42 percent. Medicine can take credit for some of the increases in longevity over the last generation, but at least half of the improvement comes from nonmedical factors, such as mandatory airbags, gun locks, and the great shift of the workforce away from farms, factories, and mines into less hazardous, service sector work. Epidemiologist John P. Bunker, a world-recognized authority on the determinants of health and longevity, estimates that only about 50 percent of the 7 years of increased life expectancy at birth since 1950 is attributable to medical care.[7]

The same period saw an astonishing increase in the cost and volume of medical care. According to Harvard health-care economist David M. Cutler, in 1960 the average American 65 or older consumed an inflation-adjusted $11,495 in health care during his or her remaining lifetime. By 2000, that number had jumped to $147,054. Yet despite this elevenfold increase in health-care spending per senior, the resulting gain in life expectancy was a mere 1.7 years.[8] Measured by its "rate of return," or the extra years of human life produced per health-care dollar spent, American medicine is amazingly unproductive and inefficient.

Nor can we say that the increasing cost of health care just reflects the aging of the population. As the baby boomers slam into old age, population aging will indeed become a major source of increased demand for health care. But over the last 30 or 40 years, the percentage of population over 65 has grown only modestly, and there is broad consensus among researchers that population aging has so far been a minor factor in driving health-care costs. For example, the Center for the Study of Health System Change has found that from 1990 to 1995, spending increases due to population aging ranged from a mere 0.1 percent to 0.3 percent, primarily because baby boomers were then still relatively young.[9]

Instead, the big cause of skyrocketing health-care costs has been increasingly intensive use of technologies and treatments that, when we look at their effects on the population as a whole, have brought negligible if any improvement in public health and longevity. For example, from 2000 through 2005, American cardiologists performed more than 7 million coronary artery angioplasties, arthrectomies, and stent insertions, at an estimated cost of $170 billion. Yet only in recent years has there been any research to determine whether these procedures work any better than simple noninvasive treatments, such as aspirin or cholestoral pills, for patients with stable coronary disease. Turns out that they don't.[10]

Similarly, most patients with back pain, including those with herniated disks, do not need back surgery, as has been shown by numerous studies over the years. Yet back surgery is among the most common operations in the United States, accounting for more than $16 billion in hospital charges (excluding physicians' fees) for more than 300,000 procedures in 2004.[11] And of course, though treatment fads come and go, we're still waiting for any truly effective treatment for cancer, let alone a cure. I am grateful to this day that Robin and I instinctively resisted suggestions from her doctors that she opt for a bone marrow transplant combined with high-dose chemotherapy. In the 1990s, tens of thousands of breast cancer patients received this expensive, painful, and once-faddish treatment before "modern" medicine eventually got around to doing clinical trials to see if it works. Turns out it doesn't.[12]

Americans spend more per person on health care than any

other country, and we have very little to show for it except more medical bills and lots of ineffective, unnecessary, and even harmful treatments. The latest confirmation comes from a study published in the *New England Journal of Medicine* in 2009.[13] It found that Medicare patients in New York State see so many specialists and receive such intensity of care that their per capita cost to government is nearly twice that of Medicare patients in Hawaii. Yet for all the extra operations, pills, and consultations New York seniors receive, they have no aggregate benefits in health or longevity to show for it.

Indeed, due to their increased exposure to staph infections, medical errors, and the trauma of unnecessary surgery and overmedication, patients in institutions that spend the most per capita have worse health outcomes than in institutions that spend the least per capita. By extrapolating from such disparities in medical practice and outcomes, researchers have demonstrated that about a third of all health-care spending in the United States could be eliminated, even as the quality of health care improved dramatically.[14]

Even some Third World countries have better life expectancy than the United States, despite minuscule spending on health care. In Costa Rica, for example, total health-care expenditures per person come to just $743 a year.[15] And Costa Rica has little more than half the doctors per capita the United States does.[16] Yet compared with the United States, life expectancy at birth is one year longer for men and exactly the same for women. Moreover, though infant and child mortality rates are higher in Costa Rica, the adult population has a substantially better chance of becoming elderly there than here. In the United States, the chance of dying between age fifteen and sixty is 13.7 percent for men and 8 percent for women. In

Costa Rica, the chance is 11.89 percent for men and 7.16 percent for women.[17]

American Health Care's Unexpected Champion

And so I was eager to accept *Fortune*'s assignment and set off to discover what had gone wrong with America's health-care system and who could fix it. My assumptions going in were typical of those held by many Americans, particularly those with conservative, pro-market views and instinctive distrust of government. For example, I assumed that the biggest single cause of the American health-care crisis was that too many of us pay for most of our care using other people's money. Hadn't the big explosion in health-care cost started after the enactment of Medicare and Medicaid, along with the vast expansion of tax-subsidized employer-provided health insurance plans?

Another underexamined assumption I brought to this project was that American health care, as inequitable and inefficient as it may be, was nonetheless the most scientifically advanced in the world. Didn't tens of thousands of rich foreigners fly in desperation to the United States every year in search of treatments they could not get at home? Outside of veterans hospitals and some chronically mismanaged and underfunded "St. Elsewheres," the American health-care system seemed the envy of the world, even if it cost too much and left too many uninsured. And I believed this was true precisely because it was the least "socialized."

Yet, as I started asking experts for suggestions about who was delivering the highest-quality, most cost-effective, innovative, and scientifically driven health care in America,

I kept hearing an answer I could not believe. It contradicted all that I thought I knew about health care and medical economics, indeed, about markets and governments in general. Yet these experts backed up their assertion by pointing me to study after study, all published in prestigious, peer-reviewed journals. These, too, I found literally incredible at first. If their claim was so true and obvious, why did so few Americans know about it? Why was there no talk of it in all our health-care debates?

Yet the hardcore data were overwhelming. They were also confirmed by the testimony of ordinary patients and doctors I talked to, and eventually by the evidence before my own eyes when I started touring facilities. Moreover, when I reflected on all that Robin and I had experienced during our ordeal—the fragmented care and record keeping, the difficulty in keeping track of patients, the amount of effort devoted to gaming insurance paperwork, and above all our lack of a long-term relationship with the institutions that provided her care—it all started to make sense.

At first I was depressed by what I learned because it was so counterintuitive, so against the received wisdom of America's business class, that I knew the editors of *Fortune* would never feature it on their cover. And I was right. We agreed on a kill fee with no hard feelings. Business is business. But as I pondered the deeper implications of what I had learned, my depression lifted, and I became excited.

A solution to America's health-care crisis does exist, I realized. Better than that, you don't have to rely on mere theoretical speculations or econometric simulations to see how it might work, nor do you have to wait around for a revolution in technology. You don't even have to travel to some far-off foreign country like Sweden, or even Canada, to see it in operation.

It's already up and running, right here in America, with hospitals and clinics located in every state, plus the District of Columbia and Puerto Rico. It is, in fact, the largest integrated health-care system in the United States.

Most of its doctors have faculty appointments with academic hospitals. Over the years two have won the Nobel Prize for medicine. Its innovations have included the development of the CT scanner, the first artificial kidney, the development of the cardiac pacemaker, the first successful liver transplant, and the nicotine patch, plus many advanced prosthetic devices, including hydraulic knees and robotic arms.

Health-care quality experts also hail it for its exceptional safety record, its use of evidence-based medicine, its health promotion and wellness programs, and its unparalleled adoption of electronic medical records and other information technologies. Finally, and most astoundingly, it's the only health-care provider in the United States whose cost per patient has been holding steady in recent years, even as its quality performance is making it the benchmark of the entire health-care sector.

Though comparatively few Americans, especially among coastal elites, have any contact with it these days, and even fewer qualify for its services, its example shows that it is possible to make vast improvements in the quality, safety, and effectiveness of the health care all Americans receive, and to do so for but a fraction of what an unreformed health-care system would cost. We need only open our eyes, open our hearts, and open our minds.

ONE

....

Best Care Anywhere

When you read "veterans hospital," what comes to mind? Maybe you recall the headlines about the three decomposed bodies found near a veterans medical center in Salem, Virginia, in the early 1990s. Two turned out to be the remains of patients who had wandered off months before. The other patient had been resting in place for more than 15 years. The Department of Veterans Affairs admitted that its search for the missing patients had been "cursory."[1]

Or maybe you recall images from movies like *Born on the 4th of July,* in which Tom Cruise plays an injured Vietnam vet who becomes radicalized by his shabby treatment in a crumbling, rat-infested veterans hospital in the Bronx. Sample dialogue: "This place is a fuckin' slum!"

By the mid-1990s, the reputation of veterans hospitals had sunk so low that conservatives routinely used their example as a kind of reductio ad absurdum critique of any move toward "socialized medicine." Here, for instance, is Jarret B. Wollstein, a right-wing activist and author, railing against the Clinton health-care plan in 1994: "To see the future of health care in America for you and your children under Clinton's plan," Wollstein warned, "just visit any Veterans

Administration hospital. You'll find filthy conditions, shortages of everything, and treatment bordering on barbarism."[2]

Former congressman and one-time attorney for the Department of Veterans Affairs, Robert E. Bauman, made the same point in 1994, in a long and well-documented policy brief for the libertarian Cato Institute. "The history of the [VA] provides cautionary and distressing lessons about how government subsidizes, dictates, and rations health care when it controls a national medical monopoly."[3]

And so it goes today. If the debate is over health-care reform, it won't be long before some free-market conservative will jump up and say that the sorry shape of the nation's veterans hospitals just proves what happens when government gets into the health-care business. In 2009, the organizers of the right-wing "Tax Day Tea Party" took it up again on their Web site: "LOOK AT THE VETERANS HOSPITALS AND ALL THE PROBLEMS OUR VETS HAVE EXPERIENCED," exclaimed one teabagger. "WE MUST KEEP THE FEDERAL GOVERNMENT OUT OF HEALTHCARE."[4]

I made the same argument myself, in a book published in the mid-1990s.[5] Yet here's a curious fact that few conservatives or liberals know. Who do you think receives better health care? Medicare patients who are free to pick their own doctors and specialists? Or aging veterans stuck in those presumably filthy VA hospitals, with their antiquated equipment, uncaring administrators, and incompetent staff?

An answer came in 2003, when the prestigious *New England Journal of Medicine* published a study that used eleven measures of quality to compare veterans health facilities with fee-for-service Medicare. In all eleven measures, the quality of care in veterans facilities proved to be "significantly better."[6]

Here is another curious fact. The *Annals of Internal Medicine* in 2004 published a study that compared veterans health facilities with commercial managed care systems in their treatment of diabetes patients. In seven out of seven measures of quality, the VA provided better care.[7] A RAND Corporation study published in the same journal concluded that the VA outperforms all other sectors of American health care in 294 measures of quality.[8]

Or consider this: In 2006, a study comparing the life expectancy of elderly patients in the care of the veterans health system with elderly patients enrolled in the Medicare Advantage Program showed that the mortality rates were "significantly higher" among the latter.[9] The study found that the average male patient had a 40 percent decreased risk of death over the next 2 years if he was cared for by the VA rather than through the Medicare Advantage program. For women, chances of dying in the next 2 years were 24 percent less at the VA.[10]

It gets stranger: In 2007, the *Milbank Quarterly* published a study showing the VA outperforming Medicare, Medicaid, and commercial health care in key quality indictors, including diabetic care, control of hypertension, and preventive care such as mammography. The disparities are often stunning. For example, the VA successfully treats its patients with high blood pressure in 77 percent of cases, while the commercial health-care success rate is just 67 percent.[11]

And low-tech medicine is not the only arena where the VA excels. In the late 1990s, the VA adopted a National Surgical Quality Improvement Program that was soon imitated by private-sector surgeons, but with less than perfect results. In 2009, for example, the *Journal of Surgical Research* published a study of outcomes of coronary surgery at a VA hospital versus other hospitals. Even though the VA patients were considerably sicker on average, suffering nearly twice the rate of myocardial infarction, for example, their mortality rate after surgery was barely half that of those treated outside the VA system.[12]

Or consider what veterans themselves think. Sure, it's not hard to find vets who complain about difficulties in establishing eligibility. Many are rightly outraged that the Bush administration decided in 2003 to deny previously promised health-care benefits to veterans who don't have service-related illnesses or who can't meet a strict means test. Yet these grievances are about access to the system, not about the quality of care. Veterans groups tenaciously defend the VA health-care system and applaud its turnaround. "The quality of care is outstanding," says Peter Gayton, deputy director for veterans affairs and rehabilitation at the American Legion. The Legion lists among its top legislative priorities a bill that would entitle veterans to trade in their Medicare benefits for treatment by the VA. Its annual survey of deficiencies at the various VA facilities (and of course they exist and often create headlines) is put into context by the publication's title: A System Worth Saving.[13]

For 6 consecutive years, the VA has received the highest consumer satisfaction ratings of any public or private-sector health-care system, according to surveys done by the National Quality Research Center at the University of Michigan. In its latest comparative independent survey, done in 2006, 84.3 percent of VA hospital patients expressed satisfaction with the care they received. Only 73.6 percent of Medicare and Medicaid patients expressed satisfaction.[14] Perhaps the surest measure of the VA's performance is the number of vets who are voting with their feet: despite tightened eligibility rules and the declining population of veterans, the number of patients treated by the VA increased by 29 percent between 2001 and 2008, from 4.2 million to 5.5 million.[15]

Outside experts agree that the VA has become an industry leader in safety and quality. Dr. Donald M. Berwick, president of the Institute for Healthcare Improvement and one of the nation's top health-care quality experts, praises the VA's information technology and use of electronic medical records as "spectacular." The venerable Institute of Medicine notes that the VA's "integrated health information system, including its framework for using performance measures to improve quality, is considered one of the best in the nation."[16] The *Journal of the American Medical Association* (*JAMA*) noted in 2005 that the VA's health-care system has "quickly emerged as a bright star in the constellation of safety practice."[17] Another study published in *JAMA* finds that the VA is also distinguished by its ability to overcome racial disparities in health care by doing a much better job than other health-care providers in keeping African-American patients alive.[18]

In 2007, the prestigious British medical journal *BMJ* noted that while "long derided as an US example of failed Soviet-style central planning," the VA "has recently emerged as a widely recognized leader in quality improvement and information technology. At present, the Veterans Health Administration offers more equitable care, of higher quality, at comparable or lower cost than private-sector alternatives."[19]

The Honda of Health Care

Stranger still, all the while that the VA has been winning these encomiums, it has tightly contained its cost per patient.

Even as inflation in the rest of the U.S. health-care sector has been running in double digits, the VA is not only raising the quality, safety, and effectiveness of the care it provides, but also controlling costs. As Harvard's John F. Kennedy School of Government gushed, in awarding the VA a top prize in 2006 for innovation in government: "While the costs of healthcare continue to soar for most Americans, the VA is reducing costs, reducing errors, and becoming the model for what modern health care management and delivery should look like."[20]

Precise comparisons of year-to-year costs per patient are difficult, since the mix of patients changes over time with changes in eligibility rules and with the amount of combat American forces face. In addition, many people enrolled with the VA also receive health care elsewhere, so only estimated comparisons are possible between the VA's cost efficiency and that of other providers. But here's a suggestive statistic: After adjusting for the changing mix of patients, the Congressional Budget Office estimates that the VA's spending per enrollee grew by 1.7 percent in real terms from 1999 to 2005. Compare that 1.7 percent with Medicare's real rate of growth of 29.4 percent in cost per capita over that same period.[21]

Or consider this measure of the VA's medical efficiency. Veterans enrolled in its health-care system are, as a group, far older, sicker, poorer, and more prone to mental illness, homelessness, and substance abuse than the population as a whole. Half of all VA enrollees are over age sixty-five. More than a third smoke. One in five veterans has diabetes, compared with one in fourteen U.S. residents in general. Name any chronic disease—Alzheimer's, cancer, congestive heart failure, sclerosis of the liver—and a much higher percentage of veterans have it than do Americans in general. In recent years, the VA has also had to invest massively to meet the needs of recent combat vets suffering from traumatic brain injury, post-traumatic stress syndrome, and an extraordinary level of other mental health needs. It has had to do so even while caring for Vietnam-era veterans who are more and more beset not only with the normal chronic conditions of age, but with delayed complications now linked to exposure to Agent Orange, such as type II diabetes. Yet from 2002 to 2007, a period of intense combat for U.S. forces, during which the VA generally excluded new enrollments by vets lacking service-related disabilities, the VA's spending per patient rose no faster than Medicare's.[22]

Here's another point of comparison: The VA's average expenditure per patient in 2009 was just $7,532, including the prescription drug, dental, mental health, and long-term care benefits that have long been available to VA patients.[23] The average health-care expenditure for Americans in general, including children and people who never saw a doctor during the year, was $8,160 in 2009.[24]

You might well think that the untold story here is that the VA engages in rationing. And indeed, according to a RAND study published in the *New England Journal of Medicine* in 2006, VA patients received only about 67 percent of the care that experts believe they should get. But before you say, "I knew there was a catch," consider this: the same study found that the U.S. health-care system as a whole delivers only 54.9 percent of the treatments recommended by evidence-based medicine.[25]

Because the VA lacks any financial incentive to engage in overtreatment, it saves money by avoiding unnecessary surgery and redundant testing. But "rationing" is hardly the right word to explain the VA's cost-effectiveness. Instead, Americans who *don't* use the VA stand the greatest risk of receiving inappropriate care, ranging from doctors who fail to prescribe routine preventive measures such as flu vaccines or medicine to control hypertension to vast amounts of overtreatment. According to the same study, even Americans with $50,000 or more in family income receive lower-quality health care than do VA patients in general.[26]

What a concept! Cost containment and quality improvement go hand in hand in many industries, but in health care this combination is virtually unheard of. If the VA were a car company, it would be Honda. Today's VA produces the equivalent of well-engineered, efficient, reliable, reasonably priced cars with few defects and great safety records, using proven scientific techniques and a culture of continuously improving quality control. By contrast, if America's most prestigious hospitals were auto companies, most would build cars like an Alfa Romeo or a Renault—classy to look at, and often very innovative, but unsafe, inefficient, temperamental, ridiculously expensive, and an unwise choice of transportation in situations where your life actually depends on their not breaking down.

Take-Home Lessons

If this contrast gives you cognitive dissonance, it should. The VA, after all, is a massive bureaucracy headquartered in Washington. Its medical division alone, known as the Veterans Health Administration (VHA), employs more than 247,000 workers represented by five different unions. Even many of its doctors are organized into bargaining units. It's micromanaged by Congress and political appointees. The VA is the last place most people, including myself, would expect to find true innovation in technology or human organization, let alone a world-class exemplar of best practices in health care. As one British health-care researcher puts it with typical English understatement: "It may be somewhat ironic, to both Americans and non-Americans, that through the VHA the United States has implemented a model of integrated public-sector health care that appears, on balance, to work quite well. And therein lies perhaps the most potent message of the VHA story."[27]

The VA's performance is particularly difficult for conservatives to process. Back in 2004, when the Bush administration pushed for greater use of information technology in health care as a means of improving quality and holding down costs, it wound up choosing not some well-endowed, prestigious private hospital as the place to showcase the potential, but the Baltimore VA Medical Center. That's because, despite the administration's overall faith in market forces, it could find no private-sector hospital that could begin to match the VA's use of electronic medical records. Astonishingly, 20 years after the digital revolution, only 1.5 percent of hospitals today have integrated IT systems like the VA uses, and those that do often find their commercial software programs to be buggy and inadequate.[28] "I know the veterans who are here are going to be proud to hear that the Veterans Administration is on the leading edge of change," Bush found himself exclaiming in his remarks at the Baltimore VA Medical Center.[29] If Bush found it strange or disorienting to be saying this about the largest actual example of socialized medicine in the United States, he didn't express any curiosity about how and why it might be true.

Which is regrettable. Because the story of how and why the VA became the benchmark for quality medicine in the United States suggests that vast swaths of what we think we know about health, health care, and medical economics are just wrong.

It's natural to believe, for example, as I long did, that more competition and consumer choice in health care will lead to greater quality and lower costs, because in almost every other realm it does. That's why conservatives in general have pushed for individual "health savings accounts" and high-deductible insurance plans. Together, these measures are supposed to encourage patients to do more comparison shopping, therefore create more market discipline in the system.

But when it comes to health care, it's a government bureaucracy that's setting the standard for best practices while controlling costs, and it's the private-sector that's lagging in quality and cost-effectiveness. That unexpected reality needs examining if we're to have any hope of understanding what's wrong with America's health-care system and how to fix it.

It turns out that precisely because the VA is a big, government-run system that has nearly a lifetime relationship with its patients, it has incentives for investing in prevention and effective treatment that are lacking in private-sector medicine, including that which is underwritten by Medicare and Medicaid. As we'll see, these incentives became particularly sharp beginning at the VA's lowest moment in the late 1970s. Even as the VA faced severe budget cuts and loss of political support, the large numbers of World War II and Korean War veterans it served were then beginning to experience the infirmities of old age. VA doctors in that era found themselves dealing more and more with aging patients beset by chronic conditions such as hypertension, diabetes, and cancer, and they had to find a way to manage these diseases with dwindling resources. The happy, if unexpected, result was an explosion of organizational and technological innovation, most of it started by individual VA doctors acting on their own, that the private sector still cannot match.

During the period of the VA's transformation, chronic illnesses still affected a comparatively small share of the population as a whole but are now becoming widespread as the baby boom generation ages and as increasing numbers of younger Americans experience the consequences of obesity and sedentary lifestyle. The increase in chronic illnesses gives the story of the VA's turnaround a growing relevancy. Some 20 years ahead of their time, VA doctors felt compelled to begin developing a new, highly effective model of care stressing prevention as well as safe and effective management of chronic disease. Today, the continuing improvement of this model, which is based largely on the skillful use of information technology in both treatment and medical research, has propelled the VA into the vanguard of twenty-first-century medicine. The purpose of this book is to explain the VA's unexpected triumph and to show how to make its benefits available to all Americans.

TWO

....

Hitting Bottom

No other health-care provider in the United States has had such a scandal-filled and controversial past as the VA, and so it is no wonder that many Americans have long pointed to its example as proof that government-provided health care is a very bad idea. Yet a closer look at the checkered history of the VA reveals subtler lessons, both about how government-run institutions can and do fail and about how ordinary men and women can reinvent them—even over the objection of their bosses.

The story begins with one of the biggest political scandals in American history. One afternoon in 1923, a visitor to the White House was mistakenly sent to "The Red Room" on the second floor. Approaching the door, the visitor encountered the commander in chief with his hands around a man's neck shouting, "You yellow rat! You double-crossing bastard. If you ever . . ."[1]

The object of Warren G. Harding's wrath, so goes the story, was Colonel Charles R. Forbes. Forbes was a dashing and charismatic man, fond of playing poker and living the high life. Both Harding and, especially, his wife, it was said, found him to be great company when they first met him while on vacation to Hawaii. "Colonel Forbes was the type of man around whom women always have buzzed," explained one Harding loyalist in his memoirs.[2]

But Forbes was also the type of man who, despite being a deserter in World War I, somehow became a colonel, winning the Congressional Medal and enjoying a strong leadership role in the American Legion. And he was also the type of man who could win enough confidence from the president of the United States to be appointed to the politically sensitive and morally crucial role of heading up the newly formed Veterans Bureau, where he was tasked with organizing the health care of millions of wounded veterans of the Great War.

He was a poor choice, for he also turned out to be one of the greatest crooks ever to hold high office in the United States. By the time all the investigations were over, and Forbes had been sent off to serve hard time at Leavenworth, the total tally for his graft and flagrant waste of taxpayer dollars stood at $200 million, or about $2.1 billion in today's money. Forbes took lavish kickbacks on the various veterans hospitals he built around the country. For example, he used taxpayer dollars to pay more than five times the market value for the land on which the VA hospital in Livermore, California, still stands. For his troubles, he and a fellow partner in crime each pocketed $12,500 in kickbacks. When he wasn't touring the nation, picking out other lucrative sites on which to build hospitals, he was entertaining extravagantly and living a life of luxury in Washington, ostensibly on his government salary of $10,000 a year.

To maintain his lifestyle, Forbes plied the Veterans Bureau with trainloads of unneeded provisions, such as a 100-year supply of floor wax, which he then sold off by the trainload for pennies on the dollar in exchange for kickbacks. Boxcars filled with bed sheets, drugs, alcohol, and other hospital supplies—many desperately needed by overcrowded veterans hospitals—would arrive at the railroad siding outside the Veterans Bureau's warehouse in Perryville, Maryland, only to be reloaded out the back door almost immediately for resale as "government surplus."

Not only was Forbes's graft extraordinary, but he let down millions of Great War veterans, many of them poisoned by mustard gas and otherwise grievously wounded, thereby making a "lost generation" feel even more abandoned. Reflecting on his experience with Forbes and his cronies, Harding would later famously say, "I have no trouble with my enemies. I can take care of them. It is my friends. My friends that are giving me trouble."[3]

Routineers and Mediocrities

Yet it wasn't just scandal, but attempts to avoid scandal, that marred the veterans health system for much of its history. One of the reasons the VA would later emerge as such a rule-bound and ossified bureaucracy was that, after the example of Charles Forbes, subsequent administrators were terrified by the prospect of unauthorized spending and insider graft. The first of these was Brig. Gen. Frank T. Hines. One chronicler of the VA describes him as a "bald-pated, slightly built shipbuilding businessman who spent the next twenty-two years trying to keep the Veterans Bureau (and beginning in 1930, the Veterans Administration) from the pit of financial corruption."[4]

In 1945, muckraking journalist Albert Deutsch testified

before Congress about the type of bureaucracy Hines had created:

> He placed excessive stress on paper work. Bureaucratic procedures were developed, which tied up the organization in needless red tape. Avoidance of scandal became the main guide of official action. Anything new was discouraged: "It might get us in trouble." Routineers and mediocrities rose to high office by simple process of not disturbing the status quo. Good men were frozen out or quit. . . . The agency increasingly was controlled by old men with old ideas.[5]

After World War II, Omar Bradley, the storied "soldier's general," took over the Veterans Administration for 2 years and did much to bring its health services into the modern age. At the time, the nation's newspapers were full of headlines such as "Veterans Hospitals Called Backwaters of Medicine" and "Third-Rate Medicine for First-Rate Men." In an attempt to turn the situation around and prepare for the huge wave of returning World War II veterans, Bradley had a memorandum sent to the deans of the nation's medical schools, offering them an attractive deal. They could partner with local veterans hospitals and use their facilities to help train medical internists and residents, while also having their faculties control hiring and firing decisions.[6]

This was a fateful decision that changed the course of the VA, and of American health care as a whole. Today, an estimated 65 percent of all doctors practicing in the United States have received all or part of their training in VA facilities. The deep collaboration with the nation's medical schools also helped the VA to raise the caliber of its doctors and led to veterans hospitals enjoying much better reputations, at least among the World War II generation of veterans.

One prime example is former senator Bob Dole, who remains grateful for the prolonged treatment he received in veterans hospitals after being strafed by Nazi machine gun fire during the final weeks of World War II. He married his nurse and spoke movingly throughout his life about the men and women who helped him for over 2 years to recover from his paralysis. The VA, which also did a capable job of administering the generous educational and housing benefits extended to World War II vets under the GI Bill, enjoyed a golden moment of high public esteem.

But the moment was fleeting. By the mid-1950s, Congress was already rapidly cutting the VA's budget, causing massive layoffs. Many Korean War vets discovered they could not get into VA hospitals unless they could prove they had service-related disabilities. At the same time, a census taken in 1954 found that 65 percent of patients had been in VA hospitals for more than 90 days and that 8 percent had been in the hospital for over 20 years! Many VA hospitals remained little better than warehouses for the homeless, the infirm, and the aged.[7]

It was also true, however, that, thanks to its affiliation with medical schools, the VA continued to distinguish itself by developing many innovative medical techniques. During the 1950s, Rosalyn Yalow did her work in nuclear medicine at a VA hospital in the Bronx that would later earn her the Nobel Prize. In the early 1960s, endocrine oncologist Andrew V. Schally was doing the experiments in his lab at the New Orleans VA hospital that would make him a Nobel laureate as well. In the early 1970s, the VA became the first health-care provider in the United States to install nuclear-powered heart pacemakers.

But there were also recurring instances of veterans being subjected to medical experiments and treated as guinea pigs. As early as 1950, fourteen VA hospitals, all affiliated with medical schools, were performing radiation experiments on patients under the VA's radioisotope program. Yet, while these experiments may have advanced the cause of science, there is no record that the VA even contemplated a program for acquiring informed consent until 1958.[8]

Ironically, in the course of testing the effects of LSD in the early 1960s, the VA hospital in Palo Alto, California, gave it to a man named Vic Lovell, who enjoyed "the trip" so much that he "turned on" his friend and neighbor Ken Kesey to the psychedelic experience. Kesey got himself a job at the VA to secure his supply, eventually stealing LSD from the hospital when the trials were over. While tripping with schizophrenics in the hospital's psychiatric ward, Kesey received the inspiration, he would later say, for his masterpiece, *One Flew Over the Cuckoo's Nest*. He and his band of Merry Pranksters went on to make "acid" seem cool to a whole generation of Americans.[9]

Broken Promises

At around the same time, veterans started returning from Vietnam to an ungrateful nation. Maybe it was the lucky ones who were treated to mind-altering drugs. Not only did many returning Vietnam vets find veterans hospitals woefully underfunded and run down, many found them staffed by people they regarded as hostile. Some were house officers and doctors their own age who opposed the war and had avoided the draft by going to medical school. Others were older vets who viewed Vietnam veterans as losers and who dismissed their complaints about post-traumatic stress and exposure to chemical agents like Agent Orange as unmanly. It wasn't until 1978 that the VA even set up a registry of veterans exposed to the 19 million gallons of Agent Orange and other dioxin-laden defoliants dropped on Vietnam. It wasn't until 1991 that the VA stopped demanding that Vietnam veterans exposed to Agent Orange offer proof. And only then did the VA begin to presume, for purposes of establishing eligibility for treatment, that conditions such as diabetes and some cancers may well have been caused by such exposure.

Many Vietnam veterans were also insulted by the conditions they found in veterans hospitals. In an autobiography that later became the movie *Born on the 4th of July*, Ron Kovic, a two-tour marine who was severely injured in Vietnam, told the story of his experience in a veterans hospital in the Bronx. After describing how the hospital lacked the equipment he needed as an amputee to learn how to walk again, he quoted a young doctor's matter-of-fact explanation that it was all because of the war. "The government is not giving us money for the things we need."

The result of all these tensions, hard feelings, and strained budgets was something approaching complete institutional failure at many veterans hospitals. Part of the problem was that, thanks to improvements in combat medicine and air evacuation, many Vietnam veterans were men who would have died of their wounds in previous wars, and who were now coming home instead with severe injuries and disabilities. But that was hardly an excuse for the conditions many of them faced. Activists among the new generation of vets did everything they could to draw media and public attention to the failings of various veterans hospitals, even if it sometimes meant exaggerating how bad they were.

One of those activists was Oliver Meadows, a former commander of Disabled American Veterans and staff director of the House Veterans Affairs Committee. He would later proudly recall how he and others "literally staged specials with ABC, NBC, CBS. We staged the network spectaculars. We had major articles in *Reader's Digest, Life* magazine. They were all over the country. We had a specially tailored story written for St. Louis, for example, and the local papers would pick it up. Every VA hospital in the country was covered. We released material to those papers where the hospital was located."[10]

On May 22, 1970, *Life* published a photo essay about conditions in the Kingsbridge VA hospital in the Bronx that fixed the reputation of veterans hospitals in the post-Vietnam era. The story quoted a quadriplegic lance corporal: "Nobody should have to live in these conditions. We're all hooked up to urine bags, and without enough attendants to empty them, they spill over the floor. It smells and cakes something awful. . . . It's like you've been put in jail, or you've been punished for something." Worst of all, the lance corporal continued, were the rats.

Meadows would later say the *Life* story "was totally contrived, we helped them all the way." And indeed, according to Robert Klein, author of the 1981 book *Wounded Men, Broken Promises*, which is generally an exposé of veterans hospitals, some VA officials, and at least one veteran interviewed for the *Life* story, claimed that conditions in the various VA hospitals were actually staged by activists to make them look more awful and sensational than they really were. Yet there is also no doubt that many veterans hospitals in this era had sunk into squalor and become little better than medical slums.

During the Carter years, the VA was headed by Max Cleland, himself a Vietnam veteran and a triple amputee, who would later use his considerable political skills to become a U.S. senator from Georgia and a Democratic Party icon. Yet during his tenure at the VA, many vets came to believe that Cleland had been "fragged" by his own men in Vietnam and resented his attempts to portray himself as one of them. Furious at Cleland's refusal to acknowledge the link between exposure to Agent Orange and their subsequent cancers and disabilities, a throng of Vietnam vets came close to physically attacking Cleland in his wheel chair during a Senate hearing, taunting, "Did you lose your balls in Vietnam, too?"

The Iron Triangle

Probably the only reason the veterans' health system survived this era was the "iron triangle" of inside politics. Medical schools benefited from their access to, and in many cases, control over, veterans hospitals. The major veterans service organizations, whose leadership often wound up being appointed to high positions in the VA, wanted the system improved and expanded, not eliminated, as did the public employee unions that represented much of the VA workforce. Politicians benefited from the jobs and money the VA brought to their communities, to say nothing of "free" health care the VA provided to indigent and low-income vets who otherwise would have become a local responsibility.

Even those politicians who believed that "patriotism

should be its own reward," and who regarded the veterans hospitals as "socialized medicine" gone predictably amok, did not feel comfortable voting to close veterans hospitals and found it easy not to. To this day, the various conservative organizations that rank members of Congress count votes for veterans benefits, not as examples of supporting the welfare state, but as votes for national defense.

And so the checkered course of the VA continued. Fortunately, however, in the deepest recesses of the VA's moribund bureaucracy, a quiet revolution, initially driven by a few lowly dissidents—some idealistic computer geeks, others idealistic doctors, pharmacists, and other medical personnel—had been set in motion. It was a revolution from below that, once embraced by charismatic new leadership, would lead to the VA's becoming by the end of the century a world leader in safe, high-quality, and innovative health care. The revolution got ugly at times. At one point, a suspicious fire damaged one of the dissident's computers. Others were forced to quit or were driven into effective exile. "There were some nasty, nasty games played," recalls one participant. But in the end, not even the most entrenched plutocrats in the VA's Washington office, nor their enablers in political office, could put down the insurrection of the so-called Hard Hats, as the dissidents came to call themselves.

THREE

··

Revenge of the Hard Hats

Kenneth Dickie still shudders at the memory. One day in 1979, someone snuck into his secret office in the basement of the VA Washington Medical Center. The intruder stacked piles of patient records around Dickie's DEC minicomputer, doused them with a flammable material, and set them on fire. Smoke filled the room, but fortunately for Dr. Dickie and for the future of American health care, an alarm went off in time, and the computer he was using to build the country's first practical electronic medical record system was spared. Still, Dr. Dickie recounts today, he had to have the engine of his car rebuilt several times during this period because someone kept putting salt or sand into the gas tank.

Dickie was one of the Hard Hats who developed what is today known as the VA's VistA software program. VistA, which stands for Veterans Health Information Systems and Technology Architecture, is actually a bundle of nearly 20,000 software programs, most of which were originally written in the 1970s and 1980s by individual doctors and other professionals working secretly in VA facilities around the country. These pioneers had to do their best to hide their work from their superiors because it violated VA policy and was threatening enough to elements within the VA to provoke literal sabotage. But eventually, working without a plan and without a leader, these dissident doctors would wind up creating a wonder of "bottom-up" engineering that many experts say points the way to the future of twenty-first-century health care.

Today, after a long bureaucratic war that still leaves some of its developers congregating in online support groups, VistA has radically transformed the practice of medicine within the VA and made possible a new model of health care now being emulated around the world. This unique, integrated, publicly owned information system, written by doctors for doctors, has dramatically reduced medical errors at the VA while also vastly improving diagnoses, quality of care, scientific understanding of the human body, and the development of medical protocols based on hard data about what drugs and procedures work best.

The story of how VistA first came to be is inspirational on many levels. For one, it is a shining example of a time when the "Dilberts" of the world won and their hidebound bosses were humiliated. Indeed, one of the ironies is that if the VA's leadership hadn't been so moribund for so long, the revolution that led to VistA would probably never have happened. A more "with it" leadership at the VA probably would have contracted out with some private software developer to provide its information systems. The most likely result would have been computer programs imposed on, instead of created by, doctors and other medical professionals, costing billions of dollars and written in a buggy proprietary code that ordinary users would have no ability to improve, modify, or integrate.

This story is familiar in the world of American health care, where what few electronic medical information systems are in place often inspire resistance and fail. That's what happened, for example, at Cedars-Sinai Medical Center in Los Angeles, which in 2003 turned off its brand-new, computerized physician order entry system. Doctors complained that it took 5 minutes or more to log into the system and to enter the patient and medication data needed to fill a prescription. At least six other hospitals have shut down computerized drug dispensing systems in recent years.[1]

But precisely because of its ossified traditions, the VA avoided this path. When its management failed to deliver workable information technology, the happy, if unintended, result was that various VA employees took it upon themselves to solve their own individual programming needs. Their individual efforts eventually created a highly effective hospital information system that remains unrivaled by any healthcare software developed by the private sector.

In 2003, the Bush administration's top man at the Centers of Medicare and Medicaid Services, Thomas Scully, chastised private software developers for failing to come up with programs that could even begin to match the performance of VistA—let alone its price. VistA is "open-source" software, meaning that the code itself is free to anyone who cares to download it off the Internet, and is accessible to individuals who care to modify it for their own purposes or to improve its performance. (Check out the demo at http://www1.va.gov/ CPRSdemo.) The only function VistA can't do as well as its private-sector counterparts, at least without adding some code, is tracking patient billing. Instead, because of its origins, its focus is on patient care—something the private sector just can't seem to imitate.

Cubicle Wars

VistA's origins lie in the late 1970s. Like most large institutions of the era, the VA had committed to large, centralized, mainframe computers, such as the IBM 650 Magnetic Drum Data Processing Machine, which it had been using since the 1950s for administrative purposes. These machines were jealously guarded by a tight circle of "high priests," working out of the VA's central offices and its main computer center in Hines, Illinois, who regarded anything involving bits and bytes as their exclusive preserve.

Predictably, as with many other institutions of the time, the software these high priests wrote, or more often procured from private vendors, wasn't very good, in large part because the people who actually had to use it had little role in its development. Among the many scandals that dogged the VA in the 1970s was the poor performance of its information systems, which at one point in early 1976 completely broke down, causing 647,000 checks to veterans to go unwritten or to arrive late.[2]

Nor were the high priests, whose fiefdom was known as the Office of Data Management and Telecommunications (ODM&T), much better at developing software with medical applications. One project ODM&T embarked on, which was supposed to provide doctors with a computer system they could use in laboratories, began in 1968 and wasn't ready for deployment until 1982. Just completing the VA's seventeen-step bureaucratic process for approving new software typically took a minimum of 3 years of paper shuffling on top of whatever time the actual writing of the program required. In 1980, the high priests estimated it would take them at least

10 years to develop even a rudimentary patient treatment file that could be stored in the VA's mainframes.[3]

But as it happened, this was the dawn of the era of mini- and personal computers, and a handful of technically minded doctors sprinkled throughout the VA began experimenting with writing their own software to meet their various needs. One was Kenneth Dickie, an internist at the VA Medical Center in Washington, DC, who, in an attempt to simplify and improve his own working conditions, began working on a DEC minicomputer in the hospital's basement to develop a program that would combine lab results, patient history, and other data into a single electronic medical record. "It was unbelievably difficult to track down paper records," he recalls today, "and unbelievably difficult to track down the data I wanted in those records." In this era before laptops and wireless modems, Dr. Dickie's idea was that doctors and nurses could use a single minicomputer on each ward to update, retrieve, and print out complete patient records.[4]

Meanwhile, Gordon Moreshead and Wally Fort in Salt Lake City began developing a clinical psychology data system to use in their own facility. Bob Lushene in St. Petersburg, Florida, developed online psychodiagnostic tests; Richard Davis in Lexington, Kentucky, was writing a nutrient analysis program for the treatment of diabetics; and Joe Tatarczuk in Albany, New York, was working to computerize nuclear medicine.[5]

Two other key players were Joseph (Ted) O'Neill and Martin E. Johnson. Both had been part of early government efforts to explore the potential of information technology in the practice of medicine. In late 1977, they found a new and precarious perch within the VA's Department of Medicine and Surgery (forerunner of today's VHA) and began working out of a small office, cryptically labeled "Computer Assisted System Staff," from which they conspired to build a network of programmers within the VA who came to be known as the Hard Hats. In December 1978 in Oklahoma City, O'Neill and Johnson managed to pull off a meeting of freelancing programmers within the VA and persuaded them to write in a common, user-friendly language and to share their code. But everyone had to be careful to work under the radar of those who controlled the VA's centralized mainframes, even if it meant writing code under difficult conditions.

For example, many of the freelance programmers were forced to work on "word processors" that lacked tape drives. This was because buying a true personal computer, let alone one of the era's minicomputers, would have, as one participant relates, "set off alarm bells in the Central Office back in Washington." Programming on a Wang computer designed for secretaries made sharing information and updating software very difficult. The only ways to do it were with error-prone 300-baud modems or by physically carrying disk packs the size of cake trays from one site to another—a process some characterized as "committing portability."[6] Another key programmer, George Timson, worked out of San Francisco by remote access ("quite unauthorized and quite unpaid-for," he states) with a Massachusetts firm to develop an elegant and highly effective file-sharing protocol that would become the heart of VistA.[7]

Yet, soon enough, the Hard Hats ran into trouble from the high priests who manned the VA mainframes. Many Hard Hats were fired or demoted; others had their computers confiscated. According to Timson, in one case, in Columbia, Bob Wickizer went to lunch, and found, when he got back to his computer room, that his new PDP-11/70 [a minicomputer made by Digital] had been unplugged and was in the process of being crated. By all accounts, the machine never again processed another instruction, anywhere. The Enemy had won—or so it seemed.[8]

The "Underground Railroad"

The turning point finally came in late 1981. By then, on orders from the central office, personal and minicomputers had been ripped out and locked up in closets where doctors couldn't get to them. The VA's central office had ordered a radiology system developed by Hard Hats in Columbia, Missouri, to be shut down. It had also pulled the plug on a pharmacy system under development in Birmingham, Alabama, and another one in Albany, New York.[9] When word leaked out to academic researchers of a promising patient discharge program developed by VA employees in Oklahoma City, the central office refused even to acknowledge its existence in public.

Stunned by these developments, many doctors and other medical professionals who used Hard Hat software and saw its value at last broke out in open rebellion. The controversy, which burst into the medical trade press and caught the attention of Congress, finally caused the VA's Chief Medical Director Dr. Donald L. Custis to take a field trip to the VA's Washington medical center on North Capitol Street to see what all the fuss was about.

This facility is only 6 miles away from the VA's central office on Vermont Avenue near the White House, but in those days it was also a world away. This is where Kenneth Dickie, joined by Marty Johnson, labored secretly in the basement, developing electronic medical record software. It was also where another key ally of the Hard Hats, the late Paul Schafer, practiced surgery while also serving as executive director of the National Association of VA Physicians. When Custis arrived at the hospital, its director, A.A. Gavazzi, told him straight off that the Hard Hats enjoyed "100 percent" support from the hospital's doctors.

Custis observed all the homemade software systems in use, and also all the programs clandestinely imported from other Hard Hat strongholds around the country. These included programs that recorded drug prescriptions, printed pharmacy labels, analyzed psychological tests, maintained tumor registries, and much more. All were running on a DEC PDP 1134 minicomputer that Custis's office had expressly forbidden use of for such purposes. But despite the obvious insubordination, Custis came away impressed. "It sounds like an 'underground railway' has been at work," he was heard to say, "and doing good work."[10]

Some Hard Hats started calling themselves members of the "underground railroad" and even had business cards printed up with a drawing of a steam engine. But soon, this railroad was underground no longer. Swayed by Custis's report of what he'd seen and fed up with the recurring problems with the VA's formal computer division, the new Reagan administration's top appointee to the VA, Robert P. Nimmo, and his deputy Chuck Hagel (the future U.S. senator from Nebraska) signed off on the Hard Hats' initiatives and pulled the plug on the high priests.

Key allies in Congress, such as Rep. G.V. (Sonny) Montgomery, concurred. A conference report that would later take on historical irony noted that "any further delay in proceeding with the decentralized . . . system is not justified and will only result in VA's medical computer system falling further behind the private health-care industry."[11] Hundreds of high priests got riffed—government parlance for "laid off." And within a short while, recalls Hard Hat Richard Davis, "many highly labor intensive and error prone systems of daily operations within the VA medical centers were dismantled." The Hard Hats had won.

Fortunately, all the different programs that became VistA were written in an easy to use, common language called MUMPS that lent itself to integration and file sharing. This meant that they could all be fit together, in literally less than a week, into a central module. Eventually that module grew to include more programs so that, for example, all the different forms of care a patient received, in all different parts of a hospital, as well as in clinics, could be combined into a single electronic health record.[12]

Catching the Age Wave Early

This might not at first seem like such a big deal. Even today, the potential of electronic health records to improve the practice of medicine is only beginning to become apparent to the public, or even to many private-sector health-care providers. But individual doctors practicing within the VA were already in many ways living in the world of the future. As early as the 1970s, the population they served, which was dominated by veterans of World War II, was aging rapidly, much as the U.S.

population as a whole is now beginning to experience a rapid increase in the number of elders.

This meant that VA doctors in the 1970s, like doctors everywhere today, were seeing increasing numbers of patients beset with complicated, chronic conditions such as diabetes. These conditions, which were often accompanied by numerous comorbidities such as high blood pressure and cardiovascular disease, required constant monitoring and coordinated care involving dozens of people—specialists, nurses, radiologists, lab workers, physical therapists, counselors. The nature of these chronic diseases also demanded that patients become vitally involved in their own care, such as in measuring their own blood sugar levels, and that a system be in place for keeping track of such measurements.

The comparative frailty of the population served by the VA also made patients exceptionally vulnerable to medical errors, such as different doctors prescribing dangerous combinations of drugs. The advancing age of the veterans population also put a premium on record keeping that could quickly pinpoint who, for example, was due for a flu shot or a prescription refill. Since patients approaching the end of life often consume high volumes of expensive treatment, VA doctors and administrators also had an exceptional need for data about which of these treatments worked better than others and, indeed, about which didn't work at all.

For all these reasons and more, the environment in which VA doctors were practicing medicine in the 1970s and '80s made the value of electronic health records and other information technology easier to see than in many private health-care settings. Tellingly, Kenneth Dickie found his inspiration for developing electronic medical records while trying to contend with his caseload of VA nursing home patients in the 1970s.

A final and all-important consideration was that the VA as an institution maintained a near lifetime relationship with its patients. This meant there was a pressing institutional need to coordinate record keeping among the many different VA hospitals and clinics a veteran might use over his or her life-time. And, crucially, it meant that any improvement to the quality of care the VA could achieve through its investment in information systems would rebound to its own long-term advantage. Managing diabetic care properly, for example, meant fewer expenditures for costly amputations down the road and would even help save on nursing home costs, for which the VA was potentially liable.

By contrast, in private-sector health-care settings, where patients typically move on to another plan every few years, investment in preventing long-term complications more often than not brings no return to the institution. Thus, from a very early date, both VA doctors and administrators were far more likely than their private-sector counterparts to see the value of investing in information technology that could improve the practice of medicine.

As Timson recalls,

> by the mid-80s everybody wanted everything. We finally kind of broke out of our illegitimate status as garage opera-tions in different parts of the country and proved that we could put the pieces together. And then by the middle of the 80s we were building complete hospital information systems, using, of course, hardware that was laughably limited compared to the PC that's on your desk today.[13]

Private-sector vendors repeatedly pressured Congress to make VA doctors and technicians stop writing software. But VA doctors argued persuasively that there was no product available on the market that could compete with their own, user-made system.[14]

Since then, the growth in computer power and the emergence of the Internet, far from making VistA obsolete, has allowed it to grow still more capabilities. The original software is still in place in most facilities, but it is continually updated electronically with patches that fix bugs or add new features. Today these include electronic medical records containing X-rays, pathology slides, video views, scanned documents, cardiology exam results, wound photos, dental images, and endoscopies. The code that makes all this possible isn't elegant by today's standards, but it is stable and time-tested, and it works just the way someone trying to practice state-of-the-art medicine would want it to work. For nearly 30 years, its code has been continually improved by a large and ever growing community of collaborating, computer-minded health-care professionals, both within the VA and, increasingly, from around the world, as VistA is adopted by more and more health-care providers abroad. "The beauty of VistA," says Kreis, "is certain parts of it were not engineered in the early days in the classic top-down kind of design; it was more of a bottom-up design. What it may have lost in its engineering, it gained in its relevance."

FOUR

··

VistA in Action

One can see the legacy of the Hard Hats' triumph by visiting the Washington DC Veterans Affairs Medical Center (DCVAMC). It's an imposing structure located 3 miles north of the Capitol building. When it was built in 1972, it was in the heart of Washington's ghetto, and as one nurse told me, she used to lock her car doors and drive as fast as she could down Irving Street when she went home at night.

Today, the surrounding area is gentrifying rapidly, and the medical center, too, is not what it once was. Certain sights, to be sure, remind you of how alive the past still is here. Standing outside of the hospital's main entrance, I was moved by the sight of two elderly gentlemen, both standing at near attention and sporting neatly pressed Veterans of Foreign Wars dress caps with MIA/POW insignias. One recounted that he was a survivor of the Bataan Death March.

But, even with history everywhere, this hospital is also among the most advanced, modern health-care facilities in the world—a place that hosts an average of four visiting delegations a week from around the world. The spacious lobby resembles that of a normal suburban hospital, containing a food court, ATM, and gift shop. But once you are on the wards, you notice something very different: doctors and nurses wheeling bed tables down the corridors with wireless laptops attached. How does this change the practice of medicine? Opening up his laptop, Dr. Ross Fletcher, an avuncular, white-haired cardiologist who helped pioneer the hospital's adoption of information technology, begins a demonstration.

With a keystroke, Dr. Fletcher pulls up the medical records on one of his current patients—an eighty-seven-year-old veteran living in Montgomery County, Maryland. Normally, sharing such records with an outsider would, of course, be highly unethical and illegal, but the patient, Dr. Fletcher explains, has given him permission.

Soon it becomes obvious why this patient feels that it is important to get the word out about the VA's information technology. Up pops a chart showing a daily record of his fluctuating weight over a several-month period. The data for this chart, Dr. Fletcher explains, flow automatically from a special scale the patient uses in his home that sends a wireless signal to a modem.

Why is the chart important? Because it played a key role, Fletcher explains, in helping him to make a difficult diagnosis. While recovering from Lyme disease and a hip fracture, the patient began periodically complaining of shortness of breath. Chest X-rays were ambiguous and confusing. They showed something amiss in one lung but not the other, suggesting possible lung cancer. But Dr. Fletcher says he avoided having to pursue that possibility when he noticed a pattern in the graph generated from the patient's scale at home.

It showed that the patient had gained weight around the time he experienced shortness of breath. This pattern, along with the record of the hip fracture, allowed Dr. Fletcher to form a hypothesis that turned out to be correct. A buildup of fluid in the lung was causing the weight gain. It occurred only in one lung because the patient was consistently sleeping on one side as a way of coping with the pain from his hip fracture. The fluid in the lung indicated the patient was in immediate need of treatment for congestive heart failure, and, fortunately, he received it in time.

Laptop Medicine

VistA is also an invaluable tool in managing chronic diseases such as cancer. "In the field of oncology," explains Dr. Steven Krasnow, the hospital's chief oncologist, "following blood counts of patients over time is very important. And the ability to essentially click one box and show a graph of the patient's individual blood count has been invaluable in maintaining patient safety and providing guidance to the clinician."[1]

VistA also plays a key role in preventing medical errors. Kay J. Craddock, who spent most of her 28 years with the VA as a nurse and who today coordinates the use of the information systems at the DCVAMC, explains how. In the old days, pharmacists did their best to decipher doctors' handwritten prescription orders, while nurses, she says, did their best to keep track of which patients should receive which medicines by shuffling three-by-five cards.

Today, by contrast, doctors enter their orders into their laptops, and the computer system immediately checks any order against the patient's records. If the doctors working with a patient have prescribed an inappropriate combination of medicines or overlooked the patient's previous allergic reaction to a drug, the computer sends up a red flag and prevents the doctor from continuing until the concern is acknowledged. Later, when hospital pharmacists fill those prescriptions, the computer system generates a bar code that goes on the bottle or intravenous bag. This bar code registers what the medicine is, whom it is for, when it should be administered, in what dose, and by whom.

Meanwhile, all patients and nurses have ID bracelets with bar codes. Before administering any drug, nurses must first scan the patient's ID bracelet, then their own, and then the bar code on the medicine. If the nurse has the wrong patient, the wrong medicine, the wrong dose, or the wrong time, the computer will provide a warning. The computer will also create a report if a nurse is late in administering a dose. "And saying you were just too busy is not an excuse," says Craddock.

Craddock cracks a smile when she recalls how nurses first reacted to the system. "One nurse tried to get the computer to accept her giving an IV, and when it wouldn't let her, she said, 'You see, I told you this thing is never going to work.' Then she looked down at the bag." She had confused it with another, and the computer had saved her from a career-ending mistake—not to mention possible lethal harm to the patient. Today, says Craddock, some nurses still insist on getting paper printouts of their orders, but almost all applaud the computer system and its protocols. "It keeps them from having to run back and forth to the nursing station to get the information they need, and by keeping them from making mistakes, it helps them to protect their license." The VA has now virtually eliminated dispensing errors, while in the rest of the U.S. health-care system, dispensing errors kill some 7,000 hospital patients a year, according to the Institute of Medicine.

Speak to the young interns and residents at DCVAMC and you soon realize that the computer system is also a great aid for efficiency. At the university hospitals where they had trained, the medical residents were constantly running around trying to retrieve records—first upstairs to get X-rays from the radiology department, for example, or downstairs to pick up lab results. By contrast, when making their rounds at DCVAMC, they just flip open their laptops when they enter a patient's room. In an instant, they pull up all the patient's latest data and a complete medical record going back as far as the mid-1980s, including records of any care performed in any other VA hospital or clinic.

Along with the obvious benefits this brings in making diagnoses, it means that residents don't face impossibly long hours dealing with paperwork. "It lets these twenty-some-things go home in time to do the things twenty-somethings like to do," says Craddock. One neurologist practicing at both Georgetown University Hospital and DCVAMC reports he can see as many patients in a few hours at the veterans hospital as he can all day at Georgetown. I couldn't help but wonder if Robin and I might have experienced fewer mix-ups and better access to her doctors at Georgetown's hospital if they had had access to a program like VistA.

Today, a new feature called My HealtheVet allows individuals enrolled in the VA to access their own complete medical records from a home computer or give permission for others to do so. "Think what this means," says Dr. Robert M. Kolodner, a leading Hard Hat who helped develop the program. "Say you're living on the West Coast, and you call up your aging dad back East. You ask him to tell you what his doctor said during his last visit, and he mumbles something about taking a blue pill and a white one. Starting this summer, you'll be able to monitor his medical record, and know exactly what pills he is supposed to be taking." Through the My HealtheVet Web site, which is integrated with VistA, vets are also able to refill prescriptions and keep track of personal health information, such as blood pressure and blood sugar readings. They will also soon have the ability to make appointments online. A new pilot project with Kaiser Permanente is also under way that should eventually allow for the sharing of VistA patient records with health-care providers outside the VA even if they use a different system.

VistA also reminds doctors about patients who need to make appointments and what medications they need. For example, it keeps track of which vets are due for a flu shot, a breast-cancer screen, or other follow-up care—a task that is virtually impossible to accomplish using paper records. Today, the VA estimates that VistA has saved 6,000 lives by improving rates of pneumonia vaccination among veterans with emphysema and cutting pneumonia hospitalizations in half, thereby reducing costs by $40 million per year. At the same time, because VistA was written by VA personnel themselves, the VA pays no royalties for its use.

Another benefit of electronic records became apparent in 2004 when drug maker Merck announced a recall of its popular arthritis medication Vioxx. The VA was able to identify which of its patients were on the drug, literally within minutes, and to switch them to less dangerous substitutes within days.

That same year, in the midst of a nationwide shortage of flu vaccine, the system also allowed the VA to identify, almost instantly, which veterans were in greatest need of receiving a flu shot and to make sure they got one. One aging relative of mine—a man who has had cancer and been in and out of nursing homes—wryly reported that he beat out 5,000 other veterans in the New London, Connecticut area in getting a flu shot. He was happy that his local veterans hospital told him he qualified but somewhat alarmed by what this implied about his health. During the 2004–2005 flu season, 75 percent of all VA patients age sixty-five and over received a flu shot, as opposed to only 63 percent of Americans in that age group who were not enrolled in the VA.[3]

The VistA system also helps to put a lot more science into the practice of medicine. Its electronic medical records collectively form a powerful database that enables researchers to look back and see what drugs and procedures work better than others, without having to assemble and rifle through tons of paper records. For example, using VistA to examine 12,000 medical records, VA researchers were able to see how diabetics were treated by different doctors, hospitals, and clinics, and with what outcomes. This allowed for development of treatment protocols based on hard data, rather than, as is often the case, on factors such as where a doctor went to medical school or highly variable, local traditions of care.[4]

Wired for Science

VistA is also useful in identifying medical procedures that don't work, as well as particular doctors or surgeons who are not getting good results. For example, VA researchers have been able to use VistA's database of medical records to create the first national, risk-adjusted analysis of how patients fare after undergoing different types of surgery in different veterans hospitals. The study showed good news for the system as a whole. Between 1994 and 1998, mortality rates for major surgery fell by 9 percent, while morbidity rates, or the rate of complications after surgery, fell by 30 percent. But the study also quickly showed where outcomes were best and worst, thereby pointing to which surgical teams could stand as exemplars and which needed improvement.[5]

VistA's records can also provide important insights into the environmental factors behind disease and reveal important and otherwise overlooked correlations. For example, in October 2005, Dr. Fletcher, with a few keystrokes, checked to see how many patients in DCVAMC had blood pressure readings exceeding 140/90. The answer that came back was 45 percent. When he checked again in January 2006, he found that 50 percent had readings exceeding 140/90. Perplexed, he had VistA retrieve all blood pressure readings going back to 1998 and made an important discovery: blood pressures increase every winter and drop every summer. This insight has important implications for how blood pressure readings are interpreted and for prescribing appropriate medications. It has only come to light because of VistA.

VistA also makes it possible to track down new disease vectors with great speed and effectiveness. For example, when a veterans hospital in Kansas City noticed an outbreak of a rare form of pneumonia among its patients, its computer system quickly spotted the problem: all the patients had been treated with what turned out to be the same bad batch of nasal spray. VistA today plays a key role in the VA's avian flu surveillance program and allows for real-time data links with the Centers for Disease Control and Prevention—features that are likely to be invaluable in the event of bioterrorist attacks as well.

VistA has also proved invaluable during natural disasters. When Hurricanes Katrina and Rita devastated New Orleans and the Gulf Coast in 2005, just about the only people whose health-care records weren't gone with the wind or buried in mud were veterans enlisted with the VA, and it made a big difference. Floodwater swamped the VA hospital in New Orleans and destroyed its hospital in Gulfport, Mississippi. In all, an estimated 100,000 veterans in the area were forced to evacuate. But thanks to VistA's backup files, all patient records were preserved and within 100 hours became continuously available through a special Web site accessible to VA medical personnel around the country. "So if the patient walked into any VA and said, 'I'm an evacuee from New Orleans,'" explains Terry Algood, chief of pharmacy at the Jackson Veterans Affairs Medical Center in Mississippi, "then that meant I could call into the Katrina Web site, look at the prescriptions, and then transfer those prescriptions into their database right there and take care of the patient on the spot."[6]

The VA estimates the total direct cost of installing VistA came to about $300 million in wiring and $450 million in computers. Its upkeep costs $485 million per annum, or about $90 per patient—quite a bargain![7]

But it is not just information technology spawned by the Hard Hats that transformed the VA into what is now the nation's best-performing health-care system. It also took shrewd and charismatic leadership from above to reengineer its culture and rationalize its processes. The story of the man who led that effort is one of the few truly successful examples of the Clinton era's many attempts to "reinvent" government. In essence, he succeeded by allowing the institution to take advantage of three of its unique features: its large-scale and deeply integrated information systems, its long-term relationship with its patients, and its comparative freedom from market-driven forces that have impeded the quest for quality health care in the private sector.

FIVE

The Kizer Revolution

Thanks to the triumph of the Hard Hats, the veterans health-care system was emerging in the mid-1990s as a world leader in the use of information technology to improve the practice of medicine. But the system was in deep political crisis—a quarter of its hospital beds were empty.[1] One government audit in 1994 found that 21 out of 153 VA surgeons had gone a year or more without picking up a scalpel.[2]

It looked like what would finally undo the veterans health-care system was the rapidly declining population of veterans. By the mid-1990s, World War II veterans were passing away at a rate of 1,000 per day. Moreover, those who survived in retirement tended to migrate from the Northeast and the Midwest to the Sunbelt, leaving veterans hospitals in places like Pittsburgh or on the Colorado plains with wards of empty beds and idle staff. Meanwhile, in places like Tampa and St. Petersburg, veterans hospitals were overwhelmed with new patients, who, facing overcrowded conditions and overworked staff, found plenty to complain about.

Adding to the threatening climate of opinion, some liberals as well as conservatives were beginning to ask questions about the veterans health-care system that they would not have dared to raise at any other time in the twentieth century. "You mention the word 'veteran,' and you're supposed to pitch forward on your sword," Senator Alan K. Simpson, Republican of Wyoming and chairman of the Veterans' Affairs Committee, complained to the *New York Times* in 1994. He and other fiscal hawks increasingly saw spending on veterans health as just another wasteful form of pork barrel spending.

Meanwhile, serious voices on the other end of the political spectrum called for simply dismantling the veterans health system. Richard Cogan, a senior fellow at the Center on Budget and Policy Priorities in Washington, told the *New York Times* in 1996: "The real question is whether there should be a veterans health-care system at all."[3] At a time when the other health-care systems were expanding outpatient clinics, the VA still required hospital stays for routine operations like cataract surgery. A patient couldn't even receive a pair of crutches without checking in. Its management system was so ossified and top-down that permission for such trivial expenditures as $9.82 for a computer cable had to be approved in Washington at the highest levels of the bureaucracy.[4]

The major veterans service organizations, such as the American Legion, still supported the VA, but many individual veterans, especially younger ones, would use its hospitals only as a last resort. Hollywood once again captured and helped reinforce the public's negative perception of the VA with the movie *Article 99*, which was about a group of doctors in a veterans hospital who had to contend with too many patients, budget cuts, and ruthless administrators.

Press reports, meanwhile, continued to serve up chilling anecdotes and damning conclusions. "The VA's War on

Health" read a *Wall Street Journal* headline in 1993. "The Worst Health Care in the Nation," the *Washington Times* echoed in 1994. It was a demoralizing time for those who still believed in the nobility of the VA's motto, which is, in words borrowed from Abraham Lincoln's second inaugural address, "to care for him who shall have borne the battle, and for his widow, and his orphan."

Within the Clinton White House, skepticism about the veterans health system also ran deep. Early in the first term, Hillary Clinton and other proponents of the administration's original health-care plan had imagined that veterans hospitals might simply be folded into a much larger federally organized system of "alliances" they were planning. Even after their master plan crashed and burned in 1993, many in the administration still questioned whether veterans hospitals ought to have a future.

Enter Ken Kizer

In January 1994, Kenneth W. Kizer, MD, MPH, was surprised to learn, if for no other reason than that he was a registered Republican, that he was on the administration's short list of candidates to head the Veterans Health Administration—a position that had remained unfilled since Clinton's election in 1992. He could hardly be sure at first what the administration might have in mind. "There were a fair number of people who thought the system wasn't salvageable: people in the administration, people out of the administration, the health policy wonks. You know, there were a fair number who just said no," Kizer recalls.

Yet his background, temperament, and intellect had given

Kizer a unique vision of not only how to reform the veterans health system, but how to turn it into a model of twenty-first century health care—a vision that fortunately reached the administration's ears. In announcing his new VA undersecretary for health, the president enthusiastically noted, "Dr. Kizer brings a wide range of clinical and administrative expertise to the VA at a time when tested leadership will be crucial to the Department's success in the framework of national health-care reform." It was a prediction that has become more true today than Clinton probably dared to imagine. Indeed, future historians may well record that among Clinton's greatest legacies was the reform of the VA, which transformed it from one of the biggest arguments against socialized medicine into one of the best arguments for it.

Kizer was idealistic enough about his vision that when he got the nod from the Clintons, he gave up a comfortable professorship at the University of Southern California, left his wife and kids behind, and threw himself into his new job. "Everyone said don't take the job. Or take it if you want to have yourself a fling in Washington, but don't delude yourself by thinking that you're actually going to be able to do anything," Kizer recalls. "There was universal consensus that if there was one agency that was the most politically hidebound and sclerotic, it's the VA. But what I saw, and what I thought the opportunity was, was that they had all the pieces."

Whatever else it was, the VA's health-care system was a *system*, however ill-fitted its various pieces might be. It operated 159 medical centers around the country, 375 ambulatory clinics, 133 nursing homes, 39 domiciliaries offering care to the homeless and substance abusers, and 202 readjustment counseling centers. Moreover, it had a clearly defined base

of patients with whom it maintained nearly lifelong relationships, thereby opening up the prospect of effective investment in prevention and disease management.

Kizer also liked VA's clear mission—to keep patients
healthy—and that it didn't have to maximize shareholders'
profits or doctors' incomes. Also, because its mission centered
on patients rather than profits, a core of VA employees were
highly idealistic and committed to improving quality. As
Kizer saw it, the great opportunity lay in truly integrating
this system and taking advantage of its potential, including
investment in prevention, primary care, and highly coordinated, patient-centered, evidence-based medicine.

Kizer was not deeply experienced in the ways of the VHA,
much less Washington. The Republican outsider, he was one
of very few people to ever head the VHA who hadn't come up
through its ranks. After his first day on the job ended at about
9:00 p.m., he found himself locked outside the VHA's underground parking lot and spent an hour pounding on doors
trying to get someone to help him retrieve his car. When he
finally did gain entry, he found his car vandalized. Weirdly,
someone had stolen the headrests.

But Kizer was well prepared in every other respect.
Orphaned at an early age, he had worked his way up through
Stanford and the University of California at Los Angeles,
becoming board certified in six medical specialties. His experience with military medicine included an internship at a
VA hospital as well as service as a rescue diver in the navy
reserves during the 1970s.

Adding to this background was Kizer's academic and professional experience in public health. He practiced emergency
medicine early in his career but says he was frustrated by the

limitations of having to care for one patient at a time. Hoping to take a more systematic and preventive approach to health care, he joined California's public health department in 1984 and rose through the ranks quickly. By age thirty-two he was appointed by California's Republican governor, George Deukmejian, to become the youngest person ever to head the department.

Developing the state's response to the new AIDS crisis was one of the responsibilities Kizer took on in that position. He also spearheaded California's toxic waste cleanup efforts and early antismoking initiatives. The latter included banning smoking for the first time in the public health department's own buildings, which proved sensitive. As it happened, California's public health department was highly unionized. Sixteen different bargaining units included everyone from its scientists to the blind vendors who sold cigarettes in the lobby. Kizer's experience negotiating with all these bargaining units would later prove invaluable at the VHA, whose workforce is represented by five different unions. But equally important was the cast of mind that accompanies a responsibility for the health of whole populations as opposed to one patient after another.

This cast of mind tends to see health care as a system, not just a collection of individual doctors treating individual patients. Thus, eliminating medical errors becomes a matter not of finding a doctor or nurse to blame but of finding root causes of failure in a health-care system's various processes and procedures, or the lack thereof. Similarly, this cast of mind naturally looks for data to answer basic questions that too often don't get asked in the day-to-day practice of medicine, such as which drugs work better than others for most people most of the time. Because they concern themselves with how health care works at the population level, people grounded in the public health paradigm also tend to see health itself as overwhelmingly determined by environmental and behavioral factors. The ecology of health, in this view, includes obvious factors like smoking or lack of exercise, but also less obvious ones, such as how much patients become involved in their own treatment, or how integrated and coordinated is the care they receive.

By the time Kizer arrived at the VHA, he was well prepared to appreciate the potential of the new systematic and data-driven model of care that was already being made possible by the development of VistA. He was also well prepared to see the necessity of reorienting the VHA away from a system that emphasized acute care delivered in hospitals by specialists and toward one that put overwhelming emphasis on prevention and patient-centered management of chronic conditions. The declining population of veterans would force the VHA to undergo painful downsizing, but in Kizer's vision this change could also be the catalyst for implementing a new and profoundly more efficient and effective model of health care.

To achieve this vision, Kizer first had to deal with politics, starting with those of the VHA itself. "The basic thesis of the transformation, when I was talking about it to people within the VA, as well as outside . . . was that we have to able to demonstrate that we have an equal or better value than the private sector, or frankly we should not exist," Kizer recalls. "That didn't necessarily go down well, at least at first. But as a taxpayer, why should I pay for a system that provides poor quality, is inefficient, wastes money, and that the customers don't like?"

Demonstrating the value of the system, both to himself and to others, required formal measures or metrics of quality. By the 1990s, it had become a truism of American business that you can't manage what you don't measure. But within American health care at the time, systematic attempts to define, measure, and improve quality were highly unusual. The British, with their nationalized health-care system, had a long tradition of systematically studying the actual outcomes of different medical procedures and systems, and acting on them. But in this country, remarkably few researchers even had the concept of what is today known as "evidence-based medicine," and their work was largely ignored by health-care providers.

Nonetheless, Kizer insisted that the system measure itself against any and all benchmarks of quality for which consensus existed among health-care professionals. The metrics were somewhat crude and often measured inputs or processes rather than outcomes, but they were better than nothing. What percentage of elderly male patients received prostate cancer screening, for example, and how did this compare with their counterparts in Medicare? How many diabetic patients received treatments based on "best practices"? How long did vets have to wait to get appointments? How often did medical errors occur, and what were their patterns? How did patient satisfaction at the VA compare with that of other health-care systems?

Kizer combined such measures into a gimmicky but effective management tool he called the "value equation," which he formulated as Value = (technical quality + access + customer satisfaction + health-care status)/(cost or price). Thanks to the continuing evolution of VistA and other reporting systems, obtaining the data for this measure of cost-effectiveness would become increasingly easier, but the answers were not always pleasing or expected. For example, while it turned out that the VHA was doing a respectable job ensuring that its few aging female patients were receiving mammograms, only about 1 percent of its elderly male patients were being screened for prostate cancer.

Right Sizing

Armed with his metrics, Kizer began leading the VHA toward its transformation. One big, unpleasant, and unavoidable agenda item was how to rationalize the VHA's excess capacity. Because of the changing demographics of the veteran population and the shift to outpatient care, the VHA had scores of hospital complexes and other facilities that had to be closed for lack of patients. It wasn't only a matter of money, it was also a matter of safety. When surgeons pick up a scalpel only one or two times a year, they are bound to be out of practice, along with all of their operating team and nursing support.

To help deal with this problem, Kizer began contracting with private hospitals in areas where there were too few patients to support a veterans hospital. He also supported expanding eligibility for health benefits to veterans who were neither poor nor needed treatment for service-connected disabilities. Yet these steps were still not enough to maintain a safe volume of care at many VA hospitals. In some extreme examples, such as the veterans hospital in Grand Island, Nebraska, the average daily census of patients had dropped to just two.

A key to building enough political support to close such

institutions was negotiating an unusual agreement with Clinton's Office of Management and Budget. Under the agreement, any money Kizer managed to save by closing hospitals wouldn't simply go back to the Treasury, as under the normal rules of federal bureaucracy, but could be used by the VHA for other purposes, such as building new outpatient clinics, expanding VistA, or ensuring that every VHA patient was assigned a primary care physician. This allowed VHA employees, veterans, and other interest groups to see that much more was going on under Kizer's leadership than just ruthless downsizing.

Another key for cutting through political gridlock was Kizer's decision to decentralize, reducing the authority at VHA's central headquarters in Washington. As part of this plan, he created a series of twenty-two regional administrative districts, most of them crossing state boundaries and vested with as much power as possible in areas such as budgets and policy making. One practical advantage was simply to put VHA managers closer to those they managed and thereby create more accountability. But the measure was also politically shrewd.

For example, as chairman of the Senate's Veterans Committee, U.S. senator John D. Rockefeller IV had considerable leverage over veterans' issues and also had a particularly contentious relationship with Kizer. The senator found his state of West Virginia divided into five regional districts, all of which fell partly in other states. Because of the state's mountainous terrain, people there have always been far more likely to travel to a neighboring state than to cross the state in search of care. This plan worked well for West Virginia's veterans. But the administrative change meant that Rockefeller needed far more cooperation from veterans and politicians in other states if he wanted to save or tinker with some particular VA facility within his state.

Regionalizing the VHA power structure had other advantages as well. "It's easier to have that dialogue with real people in the community," says Kizer, "than it is with a congressional committee, where everyone wants to stand up for the flag and 'do something' for veterans, and you've got C-SPAN there hovering." Decentralization combined with the VHA's state-of-the-art information systems also meant that it became possible to hold regional administrators accountable for a wide range of performance measures, including how well they coordinated physicians, hospitals, and medical care services for a defined population within their administrative regions.

In his original blueprint for transforming the VHA, titled "Vision for Change," Kizer wrote:

> In an integrated health-care system, physicians, hospitals, and all other components share the risks and rewards and support one another. In doing so, they blend their talents and pool their resources; they focus on delivering "best value" care. To be successful, the integrated health-care system requires management of total costs, a focus on populations rather than individuals, and a data-driven, process-focused customer orientation.[5]

Kizer presented this vision as an extension of trends that were already occurring in the private sector. In this era—before HMOs and "managed care" came to be vilified—such a spin was politically savvy. But in practice, Kizer's vision went far beyond any integration done by private-sector providers, who quickly discovered that they most often lacked a "business case" for improving quality. In contrast to even the largest HMOs, the VHA could count on a relatively stable population of patients, which in turn gave it a built-in case for pursuing quality. Take, for example, the choice of drugs it uses. Many of those drugs, such as statins, which help lower cholesterol, bring about only long-term benefits to most patients—specifically, a reduced chance of one day suffering from heart attack or stroke. An HMO in which patients are constantly churning has no real financial interest in whether the particular statins it prescribes are the most effective.

For health-care providers who lack long-term relationships with their patients, even the question of whether a drug may eventually turn out to have long-term safety problems is not an urgent concern—so long as it has been approved by the Food and Drug Administration—because by the time patients begin to experience any long-term complications, they will have long since moved on to other health plans. Because of the churning of patients that occurs in nearly every American health-care system other than the VA, decision making tends to be dominated by short-term financial costs rather than by long-term benefits to patients' health.

Workhorse Drugs

Realizing the unique incentives the VA had to maximize its patients' health, Kizer set up an elaborate drug review process to establish what is known as a "formulary" of recommended drug therapies. Field investigations by VA physicians and pharmacists compared the effectiveness of new drugs with current therapies, considered any safety concerns, and decided whether the VA should include these new drugs in its formulary.

One result was that the VA would sometimes pay for pricey drugs that typically were not covered by other health-care plans, such as an expensive but effective compound used in the treatment of schizophrenia, and high-quality statins used to treat high cholesterol. "If you know you're going to have your patients for five years, ten years, fifteen years, or life," explains Kizer, "there are both good economic and health reasons why you would want to use these more expensive drugs. You have a population of patients who are at high risk for sclerotic heart disease, and you've got them for life. You make a different decision about what's on your drug formulary than you might if you knew you only had them for a year or two."

After evaluating the safety and effectiveness of different competing therapies, the VA typically settles on a few "workhorse" drugs—such as the statin simvastatin to treat high cholesterol—that become part of the VA's standard medical protocol. This exercise in evidence-based medicine not only brings health benefits to patients but also has the effect of further leveraging the VA's already considerable purchasing power over drug companies, thus allowing it to negotiate deep discounts even on the highest-quality drugs.

Predictably, many drug companies hate the power the VA has over them. They fund studies claiming to find some inadequacy in its formulary, with the usual complaint being that the VA does not include enough "new and improved" drugs. One such study, for example, published by the drug industry–funded Manhattan Institute, purported to find a two-month decline in life expectancy among VA patients because the VA formulary included a lower fraction of new drugs than those typically in use by the rest of the health-care sector[6]

Yet the independent and prestigious Institute of Medicine has debunked the claim, finding that "the VA National Formulary is not overly restrictive."[7] As the millions of Americans who took Vioxx and other COX-2 inhibitors have learned all too painfully in recent years: just because the Food and Drug Administration approves a drug doesn't mean it is a superior therapy, or even a safe one. It only means that in some short-run trials, usually financed by the manufacturer, the new drug proved more effective than a placebo.

According to William Korchik, a VA doctor who has participated in the VA's drug review process, another big benefit of this policy over the years has been avoiding dangerous drugs.

> We took a tough stand on the [COX-2] inhibitors by not putting the drug on our national formulary and requiring prescribers to complete a risk assessment tool on each patient before a COX-2 inhibitor could be provided. . . . Predictably, we were criticized up and down about our restrictiveness. But now I can say we were appropriately restrictive because there was not data [proving their safety].[8]

By 1998, Kizer's shake-up of the VHA's operating system was already earning him management guru status. His story appeared that year in *Straight from the CEO: The World's Top Business Leaders Reveal Ideas That Every Manager Can Use*. Yet the revolution he helped set in motion at the VA was only beginning, even as the rest of the U.S. health-care system fell deeper into crisis.

....

SIX

Safety First

Everyone understands that a good health-care system needs highly trained, committed professionals. They should know a lot about biochemistry, anatomy, cellular and molecular immunology, and other details about how the human body works—and have the academic credentials to prove it. But these days, if you get sick with a serious illness, chances are you'll see many doctors, including different specialists. Three-quarters of Medicare spending goes to patients with five or more chronic conditions, who see an average of fourteen different physicians annually.[1] Therefore, how well these doctors communicate with one another and work as a team becomes critical. "Forgetfulness is such a constant problem in the system," says Donald Berwick of the Institute for Healthcare Improvement. "It doesn't remember you. Doesn't remember that you were here and here and then there. It doesn't remember your story."

Are all your doctors working from the same medical record and making legible entries? Do they have a system to make sure they don't collectively wind up prescribing dangerous combinations of drugs? Is any one of them going to take responsibility for coordinating your care so that, for example, you don't leave the hospital without appropriate follow-up medication and the knowledge of how and when to take it? Just about anyone who's had a serious illness or tried to be an advocate of a sick loved one knows that all too often the answer is no.

And it's not just doctors who define the quality of your health care. All kinds of other people are also involved— nurses, pharmacists, lab technicians, orderlies, and even custodians. Any one of these people could easily kill you by performing duties incorrectly or if some aspect of the job is not properly managed with safety in mind. Modern hospitals may not produce catastrophic failures that kill thousands of people at a time. But doctors, nurses, and hospital technicians routinely deal with very dangerous technologies and powerful drugs that do kill thousands of Americans every year, albeit usually one at a time. Even a job such as changing a bedpan, if not done right, can spread deadly infection throughout a hospital. These jobs are all part of a system of care, and if the system lacks cohesion and quality control, many people will be injured and many will die.

Just how many? Nobody knows for sure, of course. One problem is a culture of cover-up that pervades health care. All individuals involved in medicine face a very real likelihood of being sued or punished by their superiors if they admit to even trivial mistakes. Given the can-do ethos of medicine, personal shame also causes many doctors and nurses to obscure mishaps or mistakes.

Then again, many of the accidents that occur in medicine go unrecognized by all involved. The elderly patient slips into dementia and eventually a coma; no one realizes that the proximate cause of her death was a pharmacist who misread a doctor's scribbled prescription. Another elderly patient succumbs to pneumonia. No one realizes that the proximate cause of the infection was an orderly who neglected to wash his hands.

But there is no doubt the number of medical mistakes is very high. In 1999, the Institute of Medicine (IOM) issued a groundbreaking study, titled *To Err Is Human*, which still haunts health-care professionals. Hospital medical records revealed that up to 98,000 people die of medical errors in American hospitals each year.[2] Subsequent findings suggest that the study may have substantially underestimated the magnitude of the problem. For example, hospital-acquired infections alone, most of which are preventable, account for an additional 90,000 deaths per year.[3] In 2007, the IOM issued a new study that found hospital patients in the United States experience an average of at least one medication error, such as receiving the wrong drug or wrong dosage, every day they stay in the hospital.[4]

On top of this are all the errors of omission. For example, there is little controversy over the best way to treat diabetes; it starts with keeping close track of a patient's blood sugar levels. Yet, if you have diabetes, your chances are only one in four that your health-care system will actually monitor your blood sugar levels or teach you how to do it. According to a RAND Corporation study, this oversight causes an estimated 2,600 diabetics to go blind every year and another 29,000 to experience kidney failure.[5]

All told, according to the same RAND study, Americans receive appropriate care from their doctor only about half of the time. The results are deadly. In addition to the 98,000 killed by medical errors in hospitals and the 90,000 deaths caused by hospital infections, another 126,000 die from doctors' failures to observe evidence-based protocols for just four common conditions: hypertension, heart attack, pneumonia, and colorectal cancer.

Why does this extraordinary loss of life go on year after year? The short answer is that, with the large exception of the veterans health-care system, few health-care providers are integrated or cohesive enough in their management and operations to promote safety and evidence-based medicine systematically.

In health care, as in all realms of life, the root cause of most accidents is not that some single person or even group of persons made a mistake, though they may have. Instead, the root cause is almost always a lack of any system or process for preventing human error or negligence. So, for example, a nurse may inadvertently kill a patient by administering a dose of potassium chloride concentrate thinking that it is liquid Tylenol or saline solution. But the root cause of the mistake was not one person's lack of diligence, though the nurse may have been tired and distracted at the time. The root cause was the fact that both bottles were made by the same manufacturer and looked alike, and there was no system for preventing a nurse from confusing them. Because of this, firing the nurse won't prevent the accident from happening again, or even reduce its chances by much. Some other nurse will eventually also be tired and distracted and will make the same mistake until there is some systematic fix that prevents it.

Full Disclosure

Long before studies like *To Err Is Human* began to appear, the veterans health system under Ken Kizer had begun to attack safety issues systematically. His first step was to convince his boss, the late VA secretary Jesse Brown, that the VA should adopt a policy of full disclosure of any medical errors. Without this policy, Kizer argued, he could not get VA doctors and other personnel to see the scope of the problem or enlist them in creating a culture of safety.

The idea carried obvious political risk. No other healthcare provider in the United States disclosed its mistakes. Kizer recalls Brown's warning to him: "If this goes south, and politically it doesn't work out, you're the first casualty." Kizer accepted those terms and announced the policy. Starting in 1997, the VA began maintaining a Patient Safety Event Registry. Reporting of medical mistakes became mandatory. At the same time, the VA promised medical personnel that it was looking for systematic solutions to safety problems, not seeking to fix blame on individuals except in the most egregious cases. The good news was a thirty-fold increase in the number of medical mistakes and adverse events that got reported. The bad news was that those numbers, despite evidence of continued under-reporting, added up to appalling totals.

According to a report released by the VA's medical inspector, the veterans health system committed 2,927 medical errors leading to 710 deaths between just June 1997 and December 1998. In addition to medication errors, the problems described by the report included surgery on the wrong body part or the wrong patient, errors in blood transfusions, patient abuse, improper insertion of catheters or feeding tubes, and a variety of other therapeutic misadventures. Other errors included losing track of 113 patients—who turned up in hospitals and nursing homes in which they were not listed—and failing to prevent 277 patient suicides.[6]

It took a while for the press to catch wind of this report, though it was a matter of public record. Kizer remembers going to Kinko's one weekend to make a copy for the *New York Times*'s Robert Pear, who had called him at home to ask about its existence. Predictably, once Pear broke the story, it generated tough headlines around the country. "VA Finds Deadly Errors at Hospitals," trumpeted the *Orlando Sentinel*. Under the headline "Killer Hospitals" the *Detroit News* editorialized: "Congress should disband the veterans health system and hand its beneficiaries vouchers or tax credits to purchase their own health care."

But many news outlets realized the broader context. The Institute of Medicine's well-publicized *To Err Is Human* report, released shortly before, gave every reason to believe that the rate of medical errors was even worse throughout the rest of the American health-care system. The VA was at least admitting to its own mistakes, and even more impressively, doing something about them. A positive *New York Times* editorial quoted the nation's top expert in health-care safety, Dr. Donald Berwick: "The Veterans Health Administration has made a more serious commitment to improving health safety than any other large system in the country."

Lessons from *Challenger*

Among the signs of that commitment was Kizer's recruitment of former air force flight surgeon, astronaut, and NASA accident investigator James P. Bagian to head up a new national center for patient safety based in Ann Arbor, Michigan. Bagian, who supervised NASA's investigation of the 1986 *Challenger* space shuttle disaster, brought with him the view that safety can only be achieved by creating systems that are, as he puts it, "fault tolerant." O-rings and other tiny parts will fail; the challenge is to find out why and when they do, and to engineer changes that minimize the consequences. Similarly, some managers will always be tempted to discount safety concerns; the challenge is to build management processes that put the burden of proof on those who argue that a flight is safe to launch rather than on those who have doubts. At the same time, "close calls" and "near misses" will happen far more than actual accidents. The challenge here is to make sure there are processes by which as many of these close calls as possible get reported and analyzed so that their root causes can be determined and future catastrophes avoided.

Such precepts have long been recognized in the world of aviation, but no one had ever attempted to apply them systematically to the world of health care. Among Bagian's key moves was to set up a system similar to those that exist within aviation whereby VA personnel could report mistakes and near misses anonymously. Given how often medical personnel not only fear blame but also feel shame when they make a mistake, the measure was essential to gathering enough data to see the patterns that were threatening safety.

Many of these patterns involve highly technical procedures that are difficult to describe in lay terms, but others are straightforward and easy to understand. For example, most people have heard about surgeons who operate on the wrong organ or limb. It happened famously to comedian Dana Carvey, who nearly died in his forties after a surgeon unclogged the wrong artery in his heart. So-called wrong-site surgery happens in about one out of 15,000 operations, with foot and hand surgeons being particularly likely to make the mistake. Most hospitals try to deal with this risk by having someone use a magic marker to show the surgeon where to cut. But about a third of the time, Bagian's safety team has found, the root problem isn't that someone mixed up left with right; it's that the surgeon is not operating on the right patient. How do you prevent that?

Obviously, VistA helps a lot. One scan of the patient's ID bracelet puts surgical orders up on the computer screen. That's one big reason why the VHA's rate of wrong-site surgery has long been far below that of the American health-care system in general. But even VistA isn't foolproof. What if someone mistyped the orders or made a mistake in coding the ID bracelet? Drawing on his previous NASA experience, Bagian developed a five-step process that VHA surgical teams now use to verify both the identity of the patient and where they are supposed to operate. Although it's similar to the check-off lists astronauts go through before blastoff, it is hardly rocket science. The most effective part of the drill, says Bagian, is simply asking patients, in language they can understand, to state (not confirm) who they are, their birthdate or Social Security number, and what they are in for.

Another safety measure taken by Bagian was equally simple and also an important lifesaver. Acting on tips from nurses, Bagian began noticing a significant number of instances in which patients were mistakenly injected with concentrated potassium chloride. This drug, which is normally used in diluted form to treat potassium deficiencies, is easily confused with sodium chloride (saline solution) or with liquid Tylenol, which comes in a similar bottle. The fail-safe solution: a policy of never allowing the concentrate to be stored in wards, backed up by barcoding of all medications.

Following in the tradition of the Hard Hats, this last measure, which is the single most important safety feature adopted by the VHA, was made possible by ordinary VHA employees acting on their own. While returning a rental car in 1992, a nurse in Topeka, Kansas, the late Sue Kinnick, saw for the first time the use of a bar code scanner. An agent used a wand to scan her car, scan her rental agreement, and then quickly sent her on her way. A light went on. "If they can do this with cars, we can do this with medicine," Kinnick later told an interviewer.[7]

With only minimal funding and management support, Kinnick joined with pharmacist Chris Tucker and fellow nurse Russ Carlson to develop the necessary software and ran a pilot project in a thirty-bed gerontological psychiatry ward by 1994.[8] Kizer says that when he got wind of this during a network managers meeting, he said, "Wow. That's pretty impressive. I need to see this." So he got on a plane and went out to Topeka, spent a day there, walked through with them how they did it, and said, "This is something we need."

Kizer had good reason to be enthusiastic. The software virtually eliminated dispensing errors. Just within the VA's Eastern Kansas Health Care System, where it was first rolled out, it wound up preventing some 549,000 errors by 2001. There was a 75 percent decrease in errors involving the wrong medication, a 62 percent decrease in errors involving wrong dosage, a 93 percent reduction in the wrong patients receiving medicine, and a 70 percent decrease in the number of times nurses simply forgot or didn't get around to giving patients their meds.[9] At the time, there was no equivalent product available from the private sector, and even today, few hospitals outside the VA have automated their drug-dispensing systems.

Meanwhile, after asking two outside consultants to evaluate VistA, Kizer had concluded that it, too, had no rival in the private sector and ordered its universal adoption. No longer would VHA physicians be allowed to handwrite prescriptions and keep notes exclusively on paper; they'd have to learn how to use VistA if they didn't already know. His decision wasn't greeted with overwhelming acclaim. Kizer estimates that between 5 and 10 percent of VHA doctors quit over the measure. But most, he says, were older specialists that the VHA no longer needed because of its new emphasis on prevention and primary care. Moreover, the promise of VistA was just too great.

Sue Kinnick's drug-dispensing software, for example, could easily be folded into VistA, and together they became a powerful tool for safety. VistA's electronic medical records take the guesswork out of whether a comatose or incoherent patient has a history of allergic reactions to penicillin or other drugs. Kinnick's computerized dispensing system, meanwhile, takes the guesswork out of what some other doctor might have meant (Celexa, Celebrex, or Cerebyx?) with a cryptic scrawl or mumbled tape-recorded notes. In short, VistA became the "killer app" for the systematic prevention of medical errors and quality improvement.

Bright Star

Of course, medical errors still do occur in the veterans healthcare system, and when they do, they are bound to make headlines. But when you see such a headline and wonder how safe veterans hospitals really are, the key question to ask is: compared to what?

Writing in the *New England Journal of Medicine* in 2005, Harvard's Lucian L. Leape and Donald Berwick surveyed patient-safety efforts throughout American medicine and came to rather dreary conclusions. They noted that there was no statistical evidence that the rate of medical errors was declining for the American health-care system as a whole, and that there was plenty of reason to believe that new technologies and more powerful drugs were making being a patient still more dangerous.

They despaired that there still did not exist any comprehensive nationwide monitoring system for patient safety and bemoaned the widespread denial among doctors that safety was a problem in medicine. "Why has it proved so difficult to implement the practices and policies needed to deliver safe patient care?" they plaintively asked. "Why are so many physicians still not actively involved in patient-safety efforts?" But amidst their gloom over lack of progress, they still saw hope in one shining exception.

"The Veterans Health Administration quickly emerged as a bright star in the constellation of safety practice," they wrote, citing its system-wide implementation of safety practices, training programs, and investment in safety research centers. They concluded optimistically that the rest of American health care would eventually catch up to the VHA in its use of electronic medical records and wide diffusion of proven and safe practices.[10]

But as we'll see in the next chapter, this is not likely, barring very fundamental changes in the organization and financing of American medicine. The veterans health system operates under unique incentives. It makes no money by providing unnecessary or ineffective treatments or tests.

Instead, by promoting its patients' long-term health and safety, it saves money while also gaining political support and thereby securing its future funding. Its doctors also form a self-selected population of professionals who tend to worry less about maximizing their own incomes and autonomy than about pursuing a calling. In short, the VA operates under conditions that give it a case for quality—a case that the rest of the American health-care system cannot make so long as it has little or no incentive to keep people well or make them better.

....

SEVEN

Who Cares about Quality?

Medical economist J.D. Kleinke makes a revealing comparison between casinos and hospitals. Suppose you go to Las Vegas and after winning a few bets get hooked. When you start losing, you find yourself going to the cage and converting all the money in your wallet into chips. Next you max out your credit cards. Later that night, with Lady Luck still flirting but denying you the big score, you convert your checking and savings accounts into still more chips. When these are gone twenty-four hours later, the casino happily lends you another $25,000 worth of chips, which represents 40 percent of your retirement account and 30 percent of the equity in your home. Then, sipping on yet another free scotch, you make one big last bet at the craps table and are suddenly struck by a massive heart attack.

An ambulance rushes you to the nearest hospital. What's different about your new location? For one, you've gone from an institution that knows lots about you and your past to one that knows practically, or maybe even literally, nothing. The casino, before it processed your credit cards or lent you money, used advanced but routine information technology to discover details about your life, such as your current employer, whether you've been caught at or suspected of cheating in another casino, your bank account balances, whether there are liens on your house, and whether your life insurance is paid up. All it needed to retrieve these details was your name, Social Security number, and a modest investment in information technology.

But the hospital you arrive at clutching your chest has no ability to retrieve the information about your past that it needs to do its job—unless, of course, it happens to be a veterans hospital. Sure, a clerk can check out your insurance status by telephone, assuming you're conscious or remembered to carry your insurance card. A clerk can maybe even find out if you've met your deductible, assuming the insurance company's computers are "up." But outside the VA, only a handful of hospitals has made the investment necessary to retrieve electronically, even from its own records, the name of your primary care physician, for example, or what medications you're on, your history of allergic reactions to various drugs, or even the name of your next of kin. Nor can most health-care providers even communicate internally without relying on hand-delivered, handwritten notes, so that when an emergency room doctor scribbles out a prescription for beta-blockers, you wind up getting, well, who knows what?

Casinos invest in information technology because it helps them with the business they're in, which is encouraging impulsive gambling. Similarly, banks have found a business case for creating a highly integrated and sophisticated network of ATMs, to the point that you can draw cash from your account across the country and around the world. Yet hospitals make no equivalent investment in information technology to help them with the business they are presumably in, which most people would say is restoring people to health. Instead, American hospitals routinely endanger their customers and kill hundreds of thousands of them by clinging to nineteenth-century information technology. The question is why?

Kleinke has an answer that is as rude as it is true. It has nothing to do with technological feasibility. As far back as the 1970s, as we've seen, amateur programmers working on VA word processors were banging out the code for the VA's proven health-care information management system. Instead, Kleinke argues, the answer has to do with health care's dirtiest of many dirty secrets: "Bad quality is good for business. And the surest road to bad quality is bad or no information."[1]

Quality Doesn't Pay

If this strikes you as too harsh, take a breath and consider. With the exception of the VA, what do most health-care providers get paid to do? Provide health? Hardly. They get paid to provide treatments, and there's a big difference. This is not to suggest that most doctors are simply profit maximizers or indifferent to your health. Many in all walks of medicine are profoundly idealistic and believe in providing the highest-quality medicine possible. But given the system under which they operate, there is only so much idealism they can afford.

That's because, according to Lawrence P. Casalino, professor of public health at Weill Cornell Medical College, "The U.S. medical market as presently constituted simply does not provide a strong business case for quality."[2]

Casalino speaks from his own past experience as a solo practitioner and on the basis of over 800 interviews he has since conducted with health-care leaders and corporate health-care purchasers. While practicing medicine in Half Moon Bay, California, Casalino had an idealistic commitment to following emerging best practices in medicine. That meant spending lots of time educating patients about their diseases, arranging for careful monitoring and follow-up care, and trying to keep track of which prescriptions and procedures various specialists might be ordering.

Yet Casalino quickly found out that his commitment to quality wasn't sustainable, given the rules under which he was operating. Nobody paid him for the extra time he was spending with his patients. He might have eased his burden by hiring a nurse to assist with all the routine patient education and follow-up care that was keeping him at the office too late. Or he might have teamed up with other providers in the area and invested in computer technology that would have allowed them to offer the same coordination of care found in veterans hospital and clinics today. Both steps would have improved patient safety and added to the quality of care he was providing. But even had he managed to pull them off, he stood virtually no chance of seeing any financial return on such investments. As a private-practice physician, he got paid for treating patients, not for keeping them well or helping them to recover faster.

The same problem exists across all health-care markets, and it's a major factor in explaining why the VA has a quality performance record that exceeds that of private-sector providers. For example, suppose a privately managed care plan follows the VA example and invests in a computer program to identify diabetics and keep track of whether they are getting appropriate follow-up care. The costs are all up front, but the benefits may require twenty years to materialize. And by then, unlike in the VHA system, the patient will likely have moved on to some new health-care plan. As the chief financial officer of one health-care provider told Casalino: "Why should I spend our money to save money for our competitors?"

Or suppose an HMO takes a more idealistic attitude and decides to invest in improving the quality of its diabetic care anyway. Not only will it risk seeing the return on that investment go to a competitor, but it will also face another danger. What happens if word gets out that this HMO is the best place to go if you have diabetes? Then more and more costly diabetic patients will enroll there, requiring more premium increases, while its competitors enjoy a comparatively large supply of low-cost, healthy patients. That's why, Casalino says, you never see a billboard with an HMO advertising how good it is at treating one disease or another. Instead, HMO advertisements generally show only healthy families.

Indeed, any health-care provider in the private sector that holds itself out as providing high-quality care for chronic conditions risks financial ruin. That's a lesson Beth Israel Medical Center in Manhattan learned after it opened a new diabetic center in March 1999. To publicize the new venture, Beth Israel convinced a former Miss America, Nicole Johnson Baker, herself a diabetic, to pose for promotional pictures wearing her insulin pump. She also posed next to a man dressed as a giant foot, a dark reminder of how poorly managed diabetes often leads to amputation.

To avoid amputation and other dire outcomes, such as blindness and renal failure, the new center adopted a model of diabetic care that rivaled the VA's in its quality. Highly coordinated teams taught patients how to check their blood sugar levels, count calories, and find the discipline to exercise, all while undergoing prolonged and careful monitoring. Within months, the center succeeded in getting the blood sugar levels of 60 percent of its patients under control—a stunning result that brought it national attention.

But the idealists who conceived this program forgot the business they were in. Health insurers would pay only piddling amounts to cover the cost of a diabetic patient seeing a podiatrist, for example, though such care is essential to reducing the risk of amputation. And insurers would pay even less for nutrition counseling, much less exercise classes. At the same time, as word of the center's excellence in diabetic care spread, patient volume increased by 20 percent a month. Soon the center was running a large deficit, and Beth Israel administrators felt compelled to shut it down. Between 1999 and 2006, three similar centers in New York folded based on the same model of care, and for the same reason. Quality doesn't pay.[3]

It's a similar story when it comes to the management of other major chronic conditions. For example, in 1995, Duke Medical Center had the bright idea of offering an integrated, supportive program for patients with congestive heart failure. Nurses regularly called patients at home to monitor their well-being and to make sure they took their medications. Nutritionists offered heart-friendly diets. Doctors shared data about their patients and developed evidence for what treatments and dosages had the best results. And it worked—at least in the sense that patients became healthier. The number of hospital admissions declined, and patients spent less time in the hospital. The only problem? By 2000, the hospital was taking a 37 percent hit in its revenue due to the decline in admissions and the absence of complications.[4] Ten hospitals in Utah had a similar experience after implementing integrated care for pneumonia.[5]

Another example is Intermountain Healthcare, a network of hospitals and clinics in Utah and Idaho that many experts have described as a model for health reform. Intermountain is inspiring. Founded by the Church of Latter Day Saints, though now operating independently, it maintains a highly idealistic culture that is focused on measurement and a commitment to evidence-based medicine. Its CEO once explained to me that because of its large market share and comparative lack of churning in its patient base Intermountain has the same incentives the VA does to invest in prevention and effective disease management. This is no doubt true to a degree, but Intermountain still winds up being punished for doing the right thing. For example, when it developed a better protocol for taking care of premature babies, it managed to reduce the use of ventilators by more than 75 percent. Yet this triumph cost Intermountain $329,000 in foregone revenue it had previously been making off inferior care.[6]

In many other realms of health care outside the VA, no investment in quality goes unpunished. Another telling example comes from rural Whatcom County in Washington State. There, idealistic health-care providers banded together to form a creative "Pursuing Perfection" initiative designed to bring down rates of heart disease and diabetes. Following best practices from around the country, they organized multidisciplinary care teams to provide patients with counseling, education, and navigation through the health-care system. They developed disease protocols derived from evidence-based medicine. They used information technology to allow specialists to share medical records and to support disease management.[7]

But a problem arose: it created many winners, but also threatened powerful interests in the local medical establishment. The initiative greatly improved public health. It also brought much more business to local pharmacies because more people were prescribed medications to manage their chronic conditions. It also saved Medicare lots of money. But because it improved the quality of health care, it reduced the revenues of the the local hospital of the county's medical specialists.[8] One group of sixty doctors at the Madrona Medical Group of Bellingham took part in the planning but chose not to participate in the program when they realized how much the project would cost them. "We were seduced by the concept," Erick Laine, Madrona's chief executive, told the *New York Times*, "but it doesn't work." An idealistic commitment to best practices in medicine doesn't pay the bills.[9]

For American health-care providers outside the VA system, improving quality, more often than not, makes no financial sense. Yes, a hospital may have a business case for purchasing the latest, most expensive imaging devices. The machines will help attract lots of highly credentialed doctors who will bring lots of patients with them. The machines will also induce lots of new demand for hospital services by picking up all sorts of so-called pseudo diseases. These are obscure, symptomless conditions, like tiny, slow-growing cancers, that patients would otherwise never have become aware of because they would have died of something else long before. If you're a fee-for-service health-care provider, investing in technology that leads to more treatment of pseudo diseases is a financial no-brainer.

But investing in any technology that ultimately serves to reduce hospital admissions, like an electronic medical record system that enables more effective disease management, is likely to take money straight from the bottom line, however much benefit it might bring to your patients and to society. Because of its fragmented, profit-driven system, the United States now lags at least a dozen years behind other advanced industrialized countries in its application of information technology to health care. In France today, every citizen over fifteen carries a Carte Vitale, a green plastic card with a small gold memory chip which contains in encrypted form the owner's complete medical records going back to 1998, including doctor visits, prescriptions, and a complete billing history. Germans carry encrypted smart-cards, which allow authorized health professionals to retrieve their complete medical histories wherever in Germany they may happen to fall ill.[10]

The only exception to the generally laggard performance in U.S. health information technology (IT) is the VA's VistA program. It's been installed in only a handful of American hospitals outside the VA, such as Midland Memorial Hospital in Texas. But it has been widely adopted by health-care systems abroad, where profit maximization isn't an issue, including the public-health systems in Finland, Germany, Egypt, Nigeria, Mexico, India, Pakistan, Uganda, and, most recently, Jordan.[11] Dr. Ian Reinecke, the man in charge of Australia's program to bring electronic medical records to every citizen, has recruited VA officials to aid in the effort, explaining to his countrymen: "the U.S. Veterans Health Administration is regarded as one of the best and most successful e-health systems in the world."[12]

Indifferent Employers

You might wonder why market forces don't drive the rest of the U.S. health-care system to keep up with the rest of the world in the use of information technology. How is it that people in Uganda, Pakistan, and Mexico enjoy the benefits of VistA, but most Americans are stuck with doctors who use nineteenth-century information technology? Aren't Americans who buy health care concerned about its quality? If Honda can win over customers and make money by selling quality automobiles, why doesn't some other company come along that does the same for health care?

It's not as if American consumers demand low-quality, dangerous, overpriced health care. If health care were like most other markets, a Honda of health care might well emerge in the private sector. But purchasers of health care usually don't know and often don't care much about its quality, so private health-care providers can't increase their incomes by offering it.

To begin with, most Americans don't buy their own health care; their employers do. How did this arrangement come about? It's not because most employers have, or have ever had, much financial interest in the long-term health of their employees or even much stake in their short-term health— unless it involves an on-the-job injury for which they might ultimately have to pay.

Before government created workers' compensation, most employers invested little or nothing in their workers' safety, much less their long-term health. In 1907 alone, various explosions and accidents killed 3,242 American coal miners, while 4,534 railroad workers also lost their lives to workplace accidents. In 1911, when New York's Triangle Shirtwaist Factory caught fire, 146 immigrant workers perished because the owners kept the doors locked to prevent pilferage. It wasn't until progressives ranging from Teddy Roosevelt to Mother Jones at last won the fight for workers' compensation that anything like a safety-first culture began to emerge in American industry.[13]

So it is quite an irony of history that Americans ever entrusted their health or their health-care system to the control of their employers, but that's what happened without anyone giving it much thought. America's employer-based health-insurance system came about during World War II when the federal government imposed wage and price controls on the economy. To get around these wage and price controls, some companies started offering workers health insurance in lieu of raises.

Soon, the group health–insurance business was flourishing. It managed to entrench itself further by winning generous tax subsidies, whose value increased as the burden of taxation borne by the rest of the economy grew. Even with these subsidies, however, it took a strong, and often militant, labor movement, and deep fear of Communism and "socialized medicine," to convince corporate America that it had better take responsibility for providing workers with health insurance. Today, as the labor movement fades in strength and militancy, fewer and fewer employers see any need to provide any health insurance at all, much less take interest in whether that insurance actually buys high-quality medicine. Today, only 69 percent of firms without union workers even offer health insurance.[14]

Worse, few employers among this dwindling number have

the wherewithal to secure high-quality health care for their workers even if they want to. A few large employers may have the staff and the market power necessary to evaluate the quality of different health-care providers and to negotiate for greater commitments to patient safety and evidence-based medicine. And a precious few do, or at least go through the motions. For example, The Leapfrog Group, an industry-sponsored organization that presses for patient safety, has done some good work but suffers from chronic underfunding. The vast majority of employers have no interest in supporting such efforts and make no effort on their own to determine, much less change, the quality of the health care they buy on their workers' behalf.

Why? Even if an employer does a cost/benefit analysis that counts, for example, the potential gain in his workers' productivity, most of those gains will likely come far in the future. Spending $500 to help a worker quit smoking may extend that worker's retirement by ten years but not make much difference in his productivity today—indeed, his loss of stimulus previously provided by nicotine may reduce his efficiency. Similarly, time spent at the company gym, regardless of its favorable consequences for long-term health, is time spent away from the desk or the assembly line today.

The hard truth is employers have little or no incentive to invest in employees' long-term health. Otherwise, all companies would have wellness programs to encourage exercise and proper diet, and they would have long ago banded together to compel health-care providers to offer more preventive services and effective disease management. As it is, most employers who provide health insurance do so because it offers them a tax-subsidized recruitment and retention tool—one whose effectiveness depends on employees having few other health-insurance options and little opportunity to evaluate the value of the health care they receive.

Those, such as Harvard Business School professor Michael Porter, who believe pressure from employers will one day force health-care providers to compete at "the right level"—that is, for value instead of price or cost-control—cannot explain why employers have not long since done so. It's a happy thought that healthy workers make for more productive workers. But the reality is that most people who meet a payroll don't think that goal is worth the cost. As a result, they either don't offer health insurance at all or show little interest in the quality of care it buys.[16]

Imperfect Information

You might also ask about employees themselves. Don't they care about the quality of their health care? Well, of course we do. But we either don't trust, or more often don't have, the information we need to determine, say, which hospital is safer than another, much less which individual doctor is more likely to perform unnecessary surgeries.

Most of us certainly know how to compare the nominal costs of different health-care plans. And we can see to what extent these plans limit access to various specialists. But there is little we can tell about the quality of care those specialists and other doctors might provide, especially before that care is actually delivered, and often even afterward.

For example, the think tank at which I am currently a fellow changed health plans again, and I was forced to find a new primary care physician. Like most Americans, I've had to do this many times before, sometimes because I moved, sometimes because I changed jobs, and oftentimes because my employer switched health-care insurers in an effort to save money. So what did I wind up doing this time?

I make my living as a "knowledge worker." And I'm certainly no innocent when it comes to using government databases, NexisLexis, or the Internet. But none of those could provide me with anywhere near enough information to make a rational decision about which particular doctor might be better than another.

With a good deal of time, money, and know-how, you can usually figure out if a doctor has been sued for malpractice or convicted of some crime. You can also tell whether a doctor is licensed and board certified. A very few insurance companies, as well as the Centers for Medicare and Medicaid Services, also allow their computer-savvy customers to glean some data on what doctors and hospitals actually charge for different procedures. You can find Web sites that list doctors who are "gay- and lesbian-friendly," Christian, or African American, which is nice to know if such categories matter to you.[18] But as for any substantive indicator of any particular doctor's quality and performance, it's pretty much a shot in the dark.

I'm somewhat embarrassed to admit that the best strategy I could come up with in choosing a new doctor was to limit my search to those who were board certified, in group practices within ten miles of my house, graduates of medical schools I had heard of, and had Web sites. This last criterion may seem silly, but I hoped it would stand as an indicator of those comfortable enough with information technology to be likely to use electronic medical records.

My strategy worked, sort of. The one time I saw my doctor, he did come into the examining room with a laptop and was personable enough. He was even more or less on time. But the new commercial software he and his practice were trying to master allowed him to write me a prescription for blood pressure medication without indicating the dosage, much to my pharmacist's bewilderment and my own consternation.

More recently, I found myself once again in the market for a primary care physician, this time because the insurance company my employer picked out for me decided it was time to drop my previous doctor and his whole group practice from its network. As of early 2010, there was only one primary care physician in the entire Washington metro area who was both in my new insurance network and listed as taking new patients. He's a sole practioner and does not return my phone calls. Because primary care physicians don't have many opportunities to overtreat patients with unnecessary surgery and expensive scans, and because they are not well compensated by insurers, there is a shortage of them and an excess of specialists.

And so we wind up making choices in health care based on whether a doctor is in the "preferred provider network" and is taking new patients. Or maybe your best friend recommended someone. Or perhaps you selected a doctor who agrees with your diagnosis and refills the Ambien prescriptions you want. We use criteria such as liking a doctor's bedside manner or the fact that all the rich people in town go to this hospital. According to a recent survey, Americans spend twice as much time researching a car or computer purchase as they do selecting a doctor, which is not surprising given the scarcity of useful information about any provider.[19] Those

of us who are truly diligent might consult rankings of different hospitals such as those published by *U.S. News & World
Report*—as Robin and I did when we needed to decide on a
cancer clinic—or consult similar Web sites. But such surveys
rely primarily on surveys of reputation—that is, on word of
mouth—and give little weight to objective, statistical measures of quality. If they did, as we'll see in the next chapter,
most of today's highest-ranking hospitals would be revealed
as among the nation's most dangerous and ineffective.

Not knowing how to judge the quality of care that doctors
provide, we place inordinate value on our ability to switch
doctors. If one disappoints us for whatever reason, we can
move on to another. "Choice of doctor" has become in most
Americans' minds the single greatest measure of the quality
of any health-care plan— a sad irony indeed since the poor
quality and fragmentation of the U.S. health-care system are
ultimately both causes and consequences of our insistence on
choice above all else.

And thus we see results like what happened in Cleveland
during the 1990s. There, a well-publicized initiative sponsored
by local businesses, hospitals, and physicians identified several
hospitals as having significantly higher-than-expected mortality rates, longer periods in the hospital, and worse patient
satisfaction. Yet not one of these hospitals ever lost a contract
because of its poor performance.[20] To the employers buying
health care in the community, and presumably to their employees as well, cost and choice counted for more than quality and
safety. Unfortunately, as we'll see in the next chapter, the cost
of this market failure in money, injury, and death can only rise
as American medicine adopts more and more expensive, complicated, and often ineffective or dangerous technologies.

EIGHT

When Less Is More

Marjorie Williams died of liver cancer in early 2005, leaving behind a bereaved husband, two young children, and a network of loved ones and admirers who filled Washington's National Cathedral to the last pew at her memorial service. Her legacies are many, including a brilliant career as a political writer for *Vanity Fair* and columnist for the *Washington Post*. Yet she will perhaps be best remembered for her sharp and revealing descriptions, written near the end of her life, of her struggle with cancer, and about what it's like to be treated for it at some of America's very "best" hospitals.

In the first two and a half years of her illness, Marjorie received treatment from thirty-two doctors in six hospitals. She and her husband, Tim Noah, also an accomplished journalist and a friend of mine, were shrewd and well connected. They consulted with many medical luminaries in search of the very best care and treatments. And yet their quest for quality in health care was as disappointing as Robin's and mine.

"My most memorable brushes have been with an eminent surgeon," Marjorie wrote in her next-to-last column for the *Washington Post*, "whose method is to stride into the examining room two hours late, pat your hand, pronounce your certain death if he can't perform an operation on you, and then snap at your husband to stop taking notes, he can't possibly follow the complexity of the doctor's thinking."

In the same column, Marjorie described another memorable moment on her journey.

> During one hospital stay, as I sat in a wheelchair outside Radiology waiting to be pushed back to my room, I began idly flipping through my chart. A young female doctor-in-training I had never seen before stopped in front of me and said, "You know, you really shouldn't be reading your chart." I thanked her for her advice and continued reading. She repeated her admonition. I explained that I was 43 and couldn't possibly read anything worse there than I had already been told by five real doctors. Upon which she actually wrested it from my grasp. (From this I learned always to go to a stall in the ladies' room when I want to read my chart.)[1]

Such anecdotes by themselves prove nothing. But Marjorie's experience helps us to visualize the reality behind a very odd truth in American medicine. Generally, the more prestigious the hospital you check into, and the more eminent and numerous the physicians who attend you, the more likely you are to receive low-quality, or even dangerous and unnecessary, care.

America's Worst Hospitals

The evidence for this assertion is as overwhelming as it is threatening to the medical establishment. The first hint of its truth came in the 1970s, when researchers John E. Wennberg and Alan Gittelsohn noticed strange patterns across regions in how doctors treated patients. By combing through old medical records, Wennberg and Gittelsohn discovered wide and seemingly inexplicable differences in how often doctors diagnosed people with peptic ulcers, for example, or in how often people received such operations as tonsillectomies.[2] In the town where Wennberg's kids went to school, Waterbury, Vermont, 20 percent of the children had their tonsils out by age fifteen; but in next-door Stowe, 70 percent of the children got tonsillectomies.[3]

Differences in socioeconomic status could not explain the contrast. Nor was it plausible to believe that the kids in Stowe were far more in need of tonsillectomies than were kids in Waterbury. The wide variation in practice patterns suggested that something besides scientific rationality was at work in deciding which patients received what care—an idea that at the time was as radical as it was novel. Doctors, after all, were supposed to be professionals who put their patients' interests before their own and who administered care according to the dictates of science.

Gradually, Wennberg and other researchers, most of them on the faculty of the Dartmouth Medical School, found clever ways to tease out what was going on, and the emerging truth was grim. For most Americans, the two biggest determinants of what kind of treatments they receive are how many doctors and specialists hang a shingle in their community and which one of them they happen to see. The more doctors and specialists around, the more tests and procedures performed. And the results of all these extra tests and procedures? Lots more medical bills, exposure to medical errors, and a *loss* of life expectancy.

This last conclusion was truly shocking, but it became unavoidable when Wennberg and others broadened their studies. They found it's not just that renowned hospitals and their specialists tend to engage in massive overtreatment. They also tend to be poor at providing critical but routine care. For example, Dartmouth researcher Elliott S. Fisher has found that among Medicare patients who share the same age, socioeconomic standing, and health status, their chance of dying in the next five years is greater if they go to a *high*-spending hospital than to a *low*-spending hospital. One reason is that patients in high-spending hospitals with lots of specialists and high technology are also *less* likely to receive many proven routine treatments.

For example, standard, evidence-based medicine has identified aspirin as a highly effective treatment for heart attack victims. Yet, in the highest-spending hospitals, only 74.8 percent of heart attack victims receive aspirin upon discharge from the hospital, as opposed to 83.5 percent in the lowest-spending hospitals. This may be one reason why survival rates for heart attack victims are actually higher in low-spending hospitals than in high-spending hospitals.

Patients in high-spending hospitals are also far less likely to receive flu vaccines (48.1 percent versus 60.3 percent) as well as such routine preventive measures as pneumonia vaccines, Pap smears, and mammograms. This general lack of attention to prevention and follow-up care in high-spending hospitals helps to explain why not only heart attack victims but also patients suffering from colon cancer and hip fractures also stand a better chance of living another five years if they stay away from "elite" hospitals and choose a lower-cost competitor. By doing so, they not only gain a better chance of receiving effective preventive and follow-up care, but they also gain a better chance of avoiding unnecessary and often dangerous surgery. Given this unexpected reality, it is perhaps not surprising that patient satisfaction also declines as a hospital's spending per patient rises.[4]

This isn't a statistical fluke. Sure, even among equally ill patients, those who are more aware of the risks of their illnesses may move closer to more prestigious and expensive hospitals. But, while that may be a small factor, the relationship between more money spent per patient and mortality exists among teaching hospitals themselves, even within the same region. And it also applies equally to patients who moved recently and to those who did not.

From evidence like this, Fisher estimates that if medical practice in the highest-spending hospitals could only be brought in line with medical practice in the lowest-spending hospitals, financial savings of up to 30 percent could be achieved in Medicare, thereby preserving the solvency of its trust fund indefinitely. And, not only would we have that happy result, but Medicare patients would receive less-dangerous and higher-quality care as well.[5]

Results like these have been repeatedly confirmed by a cascade of similar studies. Tellingly, doctors themselves seem to know instinctively the truth behind them. In 2006, when *Time* magazine had the brilliant idea of asking doctors what scared them most about being a patient, three frequent answers were fear of medical errors, fear of unnecessary surgery, and fear of contracting a staph infection in teaching hospitals.[6]

Now perhaps it becomes more evident why the VA's health system keeps coming out on top in measures of health-care quality. Although the VA is exceptional in its use of evidence-based medicine, information technology, disease management, and root-cause approach to patient safety, its superior performance is also a measure of how fragmented and ineffective its competition is. America's medical elites are very good at attracting money and prestige, and they have a huge technology arsenal with which they attack death and disease. But they have no positive medical results to show for it in the aggregate; in fact, many signs indicate that they are providing a lower quality of care than the much maligned HMOs and assorted "St. Elsewheres."

Roemer's Law

How can we possibly explain such strange findings? The beginning of all wisdom, when it comes to understanding the business of health care, is to understand that, in this realm, supply often creates its own demand. This of course seems counterintuitive and inconsistent with our experience. After you've waited two weeks to see a specialist or to have a PET scan, it is hard to imagine that there is anything but an acute shortage of medical professionals and money to equip them.

But the real reason you have to wait to see a specialist is not that there are too few of them but that there are too many. Specialists who move into a community induce demand for their services just by offering them even if their treatments provide little or no benefits, or indeed are harmful to most patients. For a similar reason, hospital beds are almost always full because their supply is so great. Add another hospital bed, and one way or another, the local health-care system will find a way to fill it. The phenomenon is known as Roemer's law, after the late health-care economist, Milton I. Roemer, who first described it in the late 1950s and early 1960s.[7]

There are two basic explanations for why Roemer's law arises. The first involves a short circuit in the normal way supply and demand adjust to one another. In most realms of the economy, demand eventually meets supply through changes in prices. If GM produces more cars than people need or want to buy, it winds up cutting prices and offering rebates until the cars are sold. Eventually, if GM can't cover its costs, it will make fewer and fewer cars, until it eventually goes out of business—or, as it happens, gets a bailout.

By contrast, health-care prices don't drop when there is excess supply. One reason is because Medicare effectively controls health-care prices. Whatever Medicare will pay for a procedure becomes the benchmark for what other insurers will pay as well. This might not be a problem if market forces determined Medicare's reimbursement rates for different procedures. But instead, it is a bureaucratic and political process that winds up setting rates and thus ensures that whatever costs the health-care system accrues collectively are covered.

So the more capacity the health-care system adds in the form of hospital beds, specialists, and high-tech equipment, the more money comes into the system. Some parts may wind up being more amply rewarded than others according to their success in influencing Medicare's rate schedules, but for the system as a whole, there is little or no check on excess supply. Instead, excess supply is absorbed through overtreatment and inefficiency. In order for a hospital to go broke and shut down under these conditions, it takes extreme mismanagement or a decline in the surrounding community that creates large volumes of uncompensated care. If Medicare reimbursement rates prove insufficient to cover the cost of one kind of treatment a hospital offers—say, managing a diabetic's care—then a hospital can divert its resources to treatments for which reimbursement rates are more lucrative, such as heart surgery or chemotherapy.

The second reason Roemer's law applies is the stunning lack of scientific knowledge about which treatments and procedures actually work. Doctors are highly trained professionals, and most are committed enough to their calling that they would never knowingly subject patients to treatments and tests that are straightforwardly and unambiguously excessive. The problem, however, is that medical textbooks are silent about what constitutes appropriate care for patients with many different illnesses, particularly for those nearing the end of life. For example, medical textbooks offer no evidence-based clinical guidelines for how often doctors should schedule such patients for return visits, when they should be hospitalized or admitted to intensive care, or what palliative care they should receive. Nor do medical textbooks offer clear guidelines, grounded in science, about when a doctor should refer a patient suffering from a specific condition to a specialist, much less when it is appropriate to order a diagnostic or imaging test.

And so we see results like these: in Elyria, Ohio, a small town near Cleveland, citizens have been receiving angioplasties at a rate of four times the national average. It turns out that nearly all these angioplasties were performed by a group practice of thirty-one surgeons in town who have exceptional enthusiasm for the operation, perhaps because it is what they

know how to do and it pays well. In the absence of any definitive protocols concerning the effectiveness or appropriateness
of angioplasties, regulators or insurance companies can do little or nothing to crack down on even such obvious examples
of overtreatment.[8]

And if the medical establishment is this much in the dark
about what might be an appropriate way to treat your disease, where does this put you? It puts you in a spot where
you can be very easily manipulated into just going along with
whatever has become the customary way of treating your disease in the local medical community. Conversely, if you have
made up your mind that you or a loved one should receive
this or that operation or should try out some drug you saw
on television or the Internet, you can probably find a doctor
who will go along with your plans. Lacking clear guidelines
about what appropriate care is, a doctor stands a very real
chance of losing a lawsuit for refusing to offer some specific
treatment or referral, especially if most other doctors in town
routinely go along with it. At the same time, doctors, unless
they're on salary, know that deferring to patient demands will
put money in their pocket.

Other dynamics are involved as well. Dr. So-and-So per-
forms a bypass operation on a patient. This invasive procedure may or may not have been the most effective way to treat
the patient; it may not have been needed at all. But the patient
believes that Dr. So-and-So saved his life and tells friends
and neighbors. Word spreads, and gets reinforced by some
other patients of Dr. So-and-So. Other doctors in the community, who have little ability to evaluate the quality of Dr.
So-and-So's work except by word of mouth, hear these reports
from their own patients, friends, and neighbors, and soon Dr.

So-and-So's reputation builds as the hottest cardiologist in town.

For local hospitals and health-care plans, this means they must compete to get Dr. So-and-So on board, come what may. No mere hospital administrator gets to point out that there is no evidence of Dr. So-and-So's treatments being effective or even safe. Why would he or she want to anyway, since Dr. So-and-So's building practice is bringing so much money to the hospital. The administrator's job is to keep Dr. So-and-So happy.

This is pretty much what happened in one notorious case, that of Shasta Regional Medical Center in the small town of Redding, California. There, two rogue cardiologists, Chae Hyun Moon and Fidel Realyvasquez Jr., headed a team that performed extraordinary volumes of unnecessary and recklessly dangerous heart operations. In the end, both would lose their licenses, and each would pay a $1.4 million fine in lieu of federal criminal prosecution. Yet for years before, their building reputations as top-notch cardiologists brought in patients from all over Northern California. In gratitude, the hospital pampered them with department chairmanships and perks. Dr. Moon even enjoyed occasional use of the hopital's emergency helicopter to fly to golf tounaments.

Our Lady of Lourdes Regional Medical Center in Lafayette, Louisiana, provides another example of how high-volume rogue surgeons can escape scrutiny for years, either because hospital adminstrators don't know, or profit from pretending not to know, how dangerous they are. At Lourdes, there were rumors for years that one of its surgeons, a Dr. Mehmood Patel, was performing vast amounts of unnecessary heart operations. Yet it wasn't until one of Patel's fellow doctors at last secretly sued him in federal court under a special whistle-blower law that the hospital revoked his admitting privileges. The hospital subsequently agreed to pay a fine of $3.8 million but still denies it had any way of knowing about the safety or effectiveness of Dr. Patel's care.[9]

As the number of specialists in a community grows, many people cut out visits to their primary care physicians altogether. Instead, they skip from one specialist to another according to what body part gives them reason to complain that day, all the while gathering more and more bottles for the medicine cabinet. Dr. Alan Leshner, member of the National Academies of Science Institute of Medicine and former director of the National Institute of Drug Abuse, estimates that 17 percent of Americans over sixty are abusing prescription drugs.

Many other patients are like "Peggy," an elderly woman profiled in a case study of the fragmented care typically delivered under Medicaid and Medicare. At age 83, Peggy went into mysterious decline, losing her appetite and eventually becoming so dizzy that she fell and injured herself in the bathroom. For a long time, she convinced herself and others that she was simply experiencing the natural consequences of aging. But when a worried son at last arranged for a comprehensive medical examination by her primary physician, it turned out she was taking four different arthritis medications prescribed by four different doctors. Embarrassed, she explained to her primary physician that she had heard of a few other doctors who were good at treating arthritis and sought them out.[10]

It's a common delusion that when one doctor or pill doesn't do the trick, maybe adding a few more to the mix will help one to feel better. As the supply of doctors and specialists increases, the culture of medicine becomes transformed. No longer is any single physician treating the whole patient or taking responsibility for coordinating a patient's care. In places such as South Florida and Manhattan, it is no longer uncommon for patients to be seen by dozens of different specialists over the course of an ailment, each of whom will happily make referrals to still more.

Over time, this pattern of care starts to seem normal to all involved. Some lonely elders even come to enjoy retelling their stories to different doctors or to those they meet in waiting rooms. It beats staying home and watching television. This fragmented form of medicine, which exists nowhere else in the world, might go on forever except that its financial costs are unsustainable, and its toll in medical errors, overtreatment, and neglect of prevention is, or ought to be, unacceptable.

What's Wrong with HMOs?

Roemer's pioneering work in documenting how supply creates its own demand in health care had a deep intellectual influence on the once idealistic movement to create health maintenance organizations. Today, many Americans view HMOs simply as organizations designed to make money by denying them care. And it's a sad fact that many HMOs have wound up doing just that, or else using clever marketing techniques to make sure they cherry-pick only young and healthy customers who are unlikely to get sick. But it is important to remember that HMOs and other forms of managed care came into existence in large measure because of a big problem that is still with us and getting worse—namely, vast amounts of poorly coordinated, dangerous, and often excessive treatment.

The original vision of those who championed HMOs was that this form of care would vastly improve the quality of American medicine and only incidentally lower its cost. Paul Ellwood, a pediatrician who more than any other single advocate built the case for HMOs, put it this way: "My own most compelling interest as a physician was in the integration of health care, quality accountability, and consumer choices based on quality first and, secondarily, price."[11]

In the late 1960s and early 1970s, a group of doctors saw two trends that worried them—a movement toward ever greater specialization and the increasing prevalence of chronic disease in an aging, sedentary population. Recognizing that this combination required a far more systematic, integrated, and scientifically driven approach to health care, they organized the precursors of what came to be known as HMOs. Specifically, they wanted an "integrated delivery system," in which "primary care" physicians would coordinate care in large, multispecialty medical group practices that would in turn be part of a system of hospitals, labs, and pharmacies. Moreover, to address the problems of overtreatment and lack of prevention, care providers would be prepaid. As Alain Enthoven, another champion of managed care, once wrote, this would give "doctors an incentive to keep people healthy."[12]

Already by this time, it was becoming apparent to those who studied the actual effects of modern medicine on the population as a whole that a new model of care was desperately needed. The crude death rate, or total number of deaths per year per 1000 Americans, was no longer declining by the

1960s. Partly this was because the fall in birthrates since the end of the baby boom years meant that children and young adults constituted a smaller share of the population. But modern medicine itself was also a factor. Its very successes were causing a pandemic of chronic disease.

How? you might wonder. Until right before World War II, it was a truism of medicine that, as the once famous medical textbook *The Principles and Practice of Medicine*, put it: "persons rarely die of the disease with which they suffer." Instead, secondary terminal infections, primarily pneumonia, carried off most patients with incurable diseases, which is why pneumonia was once characterized by medical authorities as the "old man's friend."

Then in 1937, for the first time in history, effective treatments for infection became available. The introduction of sulfa drugs, followed by the discovery of even more effective penicillin and other powerful antibiotics, radically changed the way most people aged and died. Between 1936 and 1949, the death rate from pneumonia declined from slightly under 60 per 100,000 to just 15 per 100,000. But this triumph of modern medicine came at a price. The old man's friend and other secondary infections no longer claimed as many sick patients, so more and more people were left alive and still suffering from their primary diseases while also bearing an increased risk for such chronic conditions as cancer, congestive heart failure, or the disease that came to be known as Alzheimer's.

The unexpected result was that the incidence of chronic illness exploded while mortality rates for the population as a whole stopped improving. By the 1970s, far-sighted researchers such as Johns Hopkins's Ernest M. Gruenberg started characterizing the rapid spread of chronic diseases as examples of medicine's "failures of success." Modern medicine, in a quite literal sense, was enfeebling the population. Obviously, the answer wasn't to stop using antibiotics and other modern medical techniques. But the spread of chronic disease throughout the population did call for a new model of care.[13]

At the same time, the family doctor who made house calls and knew the circumstances of his patients was passing from the scene, and no one was taking his place. The family doctor may have carried in his bag little more than a stethoscope and various vials of opiates and alcohol, but the personal attention he paid to patients had huge, and by the 1960s, increasingly well-documented, curative powers.

Professor Kerr White showed in study after study how important an intimate and long-term relationship between doctor and patient was to health. Partly this was due to reasons you would expect, but White also found that much of the benefit of such a relationship came simply from the placebo effect. The very presence of a familiar doctor laying on hands or writing a prescription gave patients hope and strengthened their will to live.

Also involved, White found, was "the Hawthorne effect." This was a phenomenon, already famous in managerial circles, that was first observed in the 1920s among women workers in a Westinghouse plant in Hawthorne, Illinois. During the course of a company study, the workers' productivity continuously increased under both good and poor working conditions. It didn't matter, for example, if they were forced to work in dim light or bright; the women kept on working harder so long as the study continued. Eventually, researchers could only conclude that the women were flattered that someone cared enough to pay close and careful attention to what their jobs were like. White demonstrated a similar effect in health care. He showed that patients in the care of a familiar and trusted physician are demonstrably more likely to modify their behavior—quit smoking, reduce drinking, take their medications—in ways that benefit their health.

Taken together, the placebo effect and the Hawthorne effect accounted for about half the benefits of all medical interventions, White showed. Armed with this insight, he went on to invent the concept of primary care and to pioneer the idea of an integrated or "managed" health-care system centered on primary care physicians. The hope was that patients in the future would not simply get lost or be ignored as they passed from specialist to specialist.[14]

Such were the highly idealistic and data-driven concerns and issues behind the emergence of HMOs. This new model of care was specifically crafted to fit the changing nature of disease in the late twentieth century and to overcome the seemingly inevitable tendency of modern medicine toward specialization and therefore fragmentation. Cost containment was to be a happy, extra benefit of improved quality, safety, and effectiveness of care.

What went wrong? Eventually, HMOs morphed into many different forms and hybrids. Some were nonprofits, others were publicly traded companies answerable to Wall Street. Some were "staff models" that put physicians on salary; others became little more than loose networks of doctors on contract. Some were run by idealists; others by shysters, crooks, and knaves. But they all had, and still have, one important common feature—a tenuous and short-term relationship with most of their patients.

By the 1990s, most people enrolled in any particular HMO

had little or no choice in the matter; they were there because their employers were trying to save money. Nor, with few exceptions, could any single HMO expand into enough markets to hold onto its customers when they moved to other areas. The combined effect was to leave HMOs with no way to recover any investment they might make in their customers' long-term health.

It didn't help that many doctors felt threatened by the growing dominance of HMOs and other managed-care providers and complained to their patients about it. Nor were the negative press and lawsuits that some HMOs attracted helpful to the industry's image. But what ultimately undid HMOs and true managed care was that, because of the constant churning of patients, they couldn't make good on their early promise to, as Enthoven put it, "keep people healthy."

With their economies of scale and aversion to overtreatment, HMOs could help keep prices down, or at least contain them better than traditional fee-for-service medicine. The overall rate of medical inflation fell sharply in the 1990s, thanks almost entirely to expansion of managed care. But because of their lack of a long-term relationship with their patients, managed care providers could not capture for themselves, nor for those they treated, the true value that this form of health-care delivery potentially offered. Many went bankrupt. Many more responded by overscheduling doctors and discouraging access to specialists even when medically justified.

Yet as we move closer to examining the lessons the VA has to offer to the rest of the American health-care system, it is important to remember that the problems that led to America's failed experiment with HMOs and managed care did not go away. Instead, they got worse, and will get worse still in the future.

Today, more than 90 million Americans live with chronic illnesses such as diabetes, cancer, and heart disease; and seven out of ten American deaths are caused by chronic illnesses. An aging population, combined with the sedentary habits of modern Americans and medicine's own "failures of success," will continue to increase the burden of chronic diseases. On our current road, the human toll from medical errors will also increase as drugs become more potent and care becomes more fragmented. As Americans grow older, more and more people will also be killed by a health-care system that fails to deliver routine preventive measures while neglecting or mismanaging chronic illnesses like diabetes. Finally, there are limits to how much Americans can pay for health care without ruining both their own finances and those of their country. For-profit HMOs are not the answer, most people would agree. Nor is the answer simply to create more subsidies so that more people can have greater access to a fragmented health-care system that is grossly inefficient, ineffective, and unsafe. So what is the answer? The last three chapters of this book point the way.

NINE

Open-Source Medicine

Many lessons can be drawn from the VA's quality transformation over the last 15 years, but among the most important are those concerning the role of information technology in twenty-first-century medicine. In this realm, as in health care generally, many paradoxes and counterintuitive realities abound, and communicating them is challenging. Some of us are knowledgeable about computers; others of us are knowledgeable about health care; few of us are knowledgeable about both. Then still more of us know little about either. The best way to proceed, then, is with concrete examples, drawn from both the VA and elsewhere, that illustrate both the promise and the peril of the ongoing merger of information technology and health care.

Start with a tale of two hospitals that have made the digital transition. The first is Midland Memorial Hospital, a 371-bed, three-campus community hospital in southern Texas. Just a few years ago, Midland Memorial, like the overwhelming majority of American hospitals, was totally dependent on paper records. Nurses struggled to decipher doctors' scribbled orders and hunt down patients' charts, which were shuttled from floor to floor in pneumatic tubes and occasionally disappeared into the ether. The professionals involved in patient care had difficulty keeping up with new clinical guidelines and coordinating treatment. In the normal confusion of day-to-day practice, medical errors were a constant danger.

This situation changed in 2007 when Midland completed the installation of a health IT system. For the first time, all the different doctors involved in a patient's care could work from the same chart, using electronic medical records, which drew data together in one place, ensuring that the information was not lost or garbled, just as in the VA. The new system had dramatic effects. For instance, it prompted doctors to follow guidelines for preventing infection when dressing wounds or inserting IVs, which in turn caused infection rates to fall by 88 percent. The number of medical errors and deaths also dropped. David Whiles, director of information services for Midland, reports that the new health IT system was so well designed and easy to use that it took less than 2 hours for most users to get the hang of it. "Today it's just part of the culture," he says. "It would be impossible to remove it."

Things did not go so smoothly at Children's Hospital of Pittsburgh, which installed a computerized health system in 2002. Rather than a godsend, the new system turned out to be a disaster, largely because it made it harder for the doctors and nurses to do their jobs in emergency situations. The computer interface, for example, forced doctors to click a mouse ten times to give a simple order. Even when everything worked, a process that once took seconds now took minutes—an enormous difference in an emergency room environment. The slowdown meant that two doctors were needed to attend to a child in extremis, one to deliver care and the other to work the computer. Nurses spent less time with patients and more time staring at computer screens. In an emergency, they couldn't just grab a medication from a nearby dispensary as before—now they had to follow the cumbersome protocols demanded by the computer system. According to a study conducted by the hospital and published in the journal *Pediatrics*, mortality rates for one vulnerable patient population—those brought by emergency transport from other facilities—more than doubled, from 2.8 percent before the installation to almost 6.6 percent afterward.

Why did similar attempts to bring health care into the twenty-first century lead to triumph at Midland but tragedy at Children's? While many factors were no doubt at work, among the most crucial was a difference in the software installed by the two institutions. The system that Midland adopted is based on software originally written by doctors for doctors at the VA. It is, with a few qualifications we need not bother with, "open-source" software, meaning the code can be read and modified by anyone and is freely available in the public domain rather than copyrighted by a corporation. For nearly 30 years, as we've seen, the VA software's code has been continually improved by a large and ever growing community of collaborating, computer-minded health-care professionals, at first within the VA and later at medical institutions around the world. Because the program is open source, many minds over the years have had the chance to spot bugs and make improvements. By the time Midland installed it, the core software, known as VistA, had been road tested at hundreds of different hospitals, clinics, and nursing homes by hundreds of thousands of health-care professionals.

The software Children's Hospital installed, by contrast, was the product of a private company called Cerner Corporation.

It was designed by software engineers using locked, proprietary code that medical professionals were barred from seeing, let alone modifying. Unless they could persuade the vendor to do the work, they could no more adjust it than a Microsoft Office user can fine-tune Microsoft Word. While a few large institutions have managed to make meaningful use of proprietary programs, these systems have just as often led to gigantic cost overruns and sometimes life-threatening failures.

And because proprietary systems aren't necessarily able to work with similar systems designed by other companies, the software has also slowed what should be one of the great benefits of digitized medicine: the development of a truly integrated digital infrastructure allowing doctors to coordinate patient care across institutions and supply researchers with vast pools of data, which they could use to study outcomes and develop better protocols.

Unfortunately, the way things are headed, our nation's health-care system will look a lot more like Children's and Cedars-Sinai (see Chapter 3) than Midland. One reason is that in the haste and panic of President Obama's first 100 days, the administration and Congress passed, as part of the so-called stimulus bill, a little-noticed $20 billion provision that deeply threatens the development of digital medicine. It disadvantages open-source vendors, who are upstarts in the commercial market. At the same time, it favors the larger, more established proprietary vendors, who lobbied for the provision. As a result, the government's investment in health IT is unlikely to deliver the quality and cost benefits the country desperately needs, and it is quite likely to infuriate the medical community. Frustrated doctors will give their patients an earful about how the crashing taxpayer-financed software they are forced to use wastes money, causes 2-hour waits for 8-minute appointments, and constrains treatment options. Done right, digitized health care could help save the nation from insolvency while improving and extending millions of lives at the same time. Done wrong, it could reconfirm Americans' deepest suspicions of government and set back the cause of health-care reform for yet another generation.

Health IT Wants to Be Free

Open-source software has no universally recognized definition. But in general, the term means that the code is not secret, is not owned, can be utilized or modified by anyone, and is usually developed collaboratively by the software's users. Does this sound familiar? Yes, the VA's underground subculture of Hard Hats was engaged in open-source software development way back in the late 1970s, though no one used the term at the time.

Today, by contrast, open-source software is quickly becoming mainstream. Windows has an increasingly popular open-source competitor in the Linux operating system. A free program called Apache now dominates the market for Internet servers. The trend is so powerful that IBM has abandoned its proprietary software business model entirely and now gives its programs away for free while offering support, maintenance, and customization of open-source programs, increasingly including many with health-care applications. Apple now shares enough of its code that we see an explosion of homemade "applets" for the iPhone—each of which makes the iPhone more useful to more people, increasing Apple's base of potential customers.

If open source is the future of computing as a whole, why should U.S. health IT be an exception? Indeed, given the scientific and ethical complexities of medicine, it is hard to think of any other realm where a commitment to transparency and collaboration in information technology is more appropriate. VistA's emergence as the world's best integrated health IT system just seals the case for open source. Yet current trends suggest that open source is not the future coming to American health-care IT.

Indeed, under the administration of George W. Bush and a Republican Congress, even the VA itself was forced to dismantle much of its open-source culture. Doing its best to recreate the dysfunctional VA of the 1970s, the Bush administration recentralized control of the VA's software development in Washington and began, in 2007, outsourcing upgrades of VistA to a proprietary software developer: the very same Cerner Corporation that botched the digitization of Children's Hospital of Pittsburgh. As a result, VistA now contains within it a proprietary "black box" controlling VA laboratory functions that no one but Cerner can modify or improve.

Under the Obama administration, the VA has committed to an open-source health IT future, yet there still have been crackdowns, in the name of security, on software programing "in the field."[1] There is reason for hope, but I have to report that the crackdowns leave some VistA software developers fuming. "This bureaucracy is under no obligation to listen to user requests," complained Frederick "Rick" Marshall in July 2009. "Instead, it listens to Congress, which listens to campaign contributors who lobby to replace VistA with their own software . . . with Congress' blessing, national development has poured most of its resources into a series of unwanted, unrealistic pork-barrel replacement projects that have squandered several billion dollars so far and left only failure, waste and demoralization behind."[2] There are signs that the Obama administration "gets" the importance of open-source health IT, but so far no definitive actions prove it.

Meanwhile, open-source communities, such as WorldVistA, and private companies, such as Medsphere, ClearHealth, DSS, and Perot System, continue modifying VistA's code for use outside the VA. In addition to the installation done at Midland, VistA is now up and running in public hospitals in Hawaii and West Virginia, as well as in hospitals run by the Indian Health Service and in many foreign countries. To date, more than eighty-five countries have sent delegations to study how the VA uses the program, even as the VA has been forced to install Cerner's proprietary software.

The partial "privatization" of health IT at the VA contains an irony that is hard to miss: private-sector development of health IT has been a colossal failure. Although health IT companies have been trying to convince hospitals and clinics to buy their integrated patient-record software for more than 15 years, only a tiny fraction of facilities have installed such systems. Part of the problem, as we've seen, is our perverse insurance reimbursement system, which essentially rewards health-care providers for performing more and more expensive procedures rather than improving patients' welfare. This system leaves few nongovernment institutions with much of a business case for investing in health IT; using digitized records to keep patients healthier over the long term doesn't help the bottom line.

But another big part of the problem is that proprietary systems have earned a bad reputation in the medical community for the simple reason that they often don't work very well. The programs are written by software developers who are far removed from the realities of practicing medicine. The resulting systems tend to create, rather than prevent, medical errors once they're in the hands of harried health-care professionals. Perversely, license agreements usually bar users of proprietary health IT systems from reporting dangerous bugs to other health-care facilities. In open-source systems, users learn from each other's mistakes; in proprietary ones, they're not even allowed to mention them.

If proprietary health IT systems are widely adopted, as is now being encouraged by government policy, even more drawbacks will come sharply into focus. The greatest benefits of health IT come from the opportunities that are created when different hospitals and clinics are able to share records and stores of data with each other. Hospitals within the digitized VA system are able to deliver more services for less, mostly because their digital records allow doctors and clinics to better coordinate complex treatment regimens. Electronic medical records also produce a large collection of digitized data that can be easily mined by managers and researchers (without their having access to the patients' identities, which are privacy protected) to discover what drugs, procedures, and devices work and which are ineffective or even dangerous. We've already seen how the VA uses VistA to monitor its own quality and the development of evidence-based protocols of care. Similarly, the IT system at the Mayo Clinic (an open-source one, incidentally) allows doctors to personalize care by mining records of specific patient populations. A doctor treating a patient for cancer, for instance, can query the treatment outcomes of hundreds of other patients who had tumors in the same area and were of similar age and family backgrounds, increasing the odds that the doctor will choose the most effective therapy.

But in order for data mining to work, the data have to offer a complete picture of the care patients have gotten from all the various specialists involved in their treatment over a period of time. Otherwise it's difficult to identify meaningful patterns or sort out confounding factors. With proprietary systems, the data are locked away in what programmers call black boxes, and they cannot be shared across hospitals and clinics. This security is partly by design; it's difficult for doctors to switch IT providers if they can't extract patient data, or if they must pay a monopolist's price to do so. In the software industry, this is known as vendor capture, the phenomenon under which users of commercial software find they cannot switch to alternative programs, because their data is locked into a secret code that only the original vendor controls. Significantly, since proprietary systems usually can't or don't speak to each other, they also offer few advantages over paper records when it comes to coordinating care across facilities. Patients might as well be schlepping around file folders full of handwritten charts.

Of course, not all proprietary systems are equally bad. A program offered by Epic Systems Corporation of Wisconsin rivals VistA in terms of features and functionality. When it comes to cost, however, open source wins hands down, thanks to no or low licensing costs. According to Dr. Scott Shreeve, who is involved in the VistA installations in West Virginia and elsewhere, installing a proprietary system like Epic costs ten times as much as VistA and takes at least three times as long—and that's if everything goes smoothly, which is often not the case. In 2004, Sutter Health committed $154 million to implementing electronic medical records in all the twenty-seven hospitals it operated in northern California using Epic software. The project was supposed to be finished by 2006, but things didn't work out as planned. Sutter pulled the plug on the project in May of 2009, having completed only one installation and facing remaining cost estimates of $1 billion for finishing the project. In a letter to employees, Sutter executives explained that they could no longer afford to fund employee pensions and also continue with the Epic buildout.

Unfortunately, billions of taxpayers' dollars are now being poured into expensive, inadequate proprietary software, thanks to the so-called HITECH provision in the 2009 stimulus package. The bill offers medical facilities as much as $64,000 per physician if they make "meaningful use" of "certi-fied" health IT in the next year and a half, and it punishes them with cuts to their Medicare reimbursements if they don't do so by 2015. Obviously, doctors and health administra-tors are under pressure to act soon. But what is the meaning of *meaningful use*? And who determines which products qualify? As of this writing, that is still not clear.

Electronic Health Record Stimulus Tour

What is clear, however, is that vendors of proprietary soft-ware are doing all they can to thwart the adoption of open-source health IT. The industry has a powerful lobby, headed by the Healthcare Information and Management Systems Society (HIMSS), a group with deep ties to the Obama admin-istration. The group is not openly against open source, but in 2008, when Rep. Pete Stark of California introduced a bill to create a low-cost, open-source health IT system for all medical providers through the Department of Health and Human Services, HIMSS used its influence to smash the legislation. The group has more recently deployed its lobbying clout to try to persuade regulators to define *meaningful use* such that only software approved by an allied group, the Certification Commission for Healthcare Information Technology (CCHIT), qualifies. Not only are CCHIT's standards notoriously lax, the group is also largely funded and staffed by the very industry whose products it is supposed to certify.[3]

Though the Obama administration is verbally committed to open-source health IT, its future is still very threatened. One big reason is the far greater marketing power that the big, established proprietary vendors can bring to bear, compared with their open-source counterparts, who are smaller and newer on the scene. A group of proprietary industry heavyweights including Microsoft, Intel, Cisco, and Allscripts has been sponsoring an Electronic Health Records Stimulus Tour, which sends teams of traveling sales representatives to tell local doctors how they can receive tens of thousands of dollars in stimulus money by buying their products—provided that they "act now." For those medical professionals who can't make the show personally, helpful webcasts are available. The tour is a variation on a tried-and-true strategy: when physicians are presented with samples of pricey new name-brand substitutes for equally good generic drugs, time and again they start prescribing the more expensive medicine. And they are likely to be even more suggestible when it comes to software, because most don't know enough about computing to evaluate vendors' claims skeptically.

What can be done to counter this marketing offensive and

keep proprietary companies from locking up the health-care IT market? Two cardiologists at the Johns Hopkins Medical Institutions, Sammy Zakaria and David A. Meyerson, recently proposed a simple solution in an op-ed piece for the *Washington Post*. They began by noting that "most currently available electronic medical record software is unwieldy and difficult to quickly access, and there is still no vehicle for the timely exchange of critical medical data between providers and facilities." The government is spending billions trying to work out the standards for a uniform record-keeping system, they further note, even though "a proven system already exists. The software is called the Veterans Health Information Systems and Technology Architecture (VistA), which the Veterans Affairs Department developed. VistA requires minimal support, is absolutely free to anyone who requests it, is much more user-friendly than its counterparts, and many doctors are already familiar with it."[4]

Seems simple, doesn't it? It is, except for the politics. Helpfully, under the Obama administration, the VA has recommitted to VistA. Its new chief information officer, Roger Baker, is on record calling VistA "the best in the world" and has said he wants to offer it to the rest of the government and the health-care industry.[5] This support is key because, unlike proprietary software, VistA has no deep-pocketed champions. Also, so long as the VA itself showed signs of wanting to abandon VistA IT, as it did when Bush's political appointees were in charge, proprietary software sales reps had a great talking point when they described VistA as a "legacy" system no longer even good enough for the VA.

Nonetheless, due to the ill-considered terms of the stimulus bill and the general power of commercial forces over U.S.

health care, this country is going to waste a lot of borrowed money on buggy proprietary software. It is too late to stop that. At least some people will get jobs installing the expensive code, and others will later be put to work pulling it out, which could count as stimulus, I guess. But what we cannot afford is to let more time pass before taking advantage of the true promise of digital health care, a precondition for which is open and uniform standards. This VistA can provide—instantly, and at no cost in royalties.

Committing to VistA as a national health IT foundation promises much more. Viewed correctly, VistA isn't a program, or even a series of programs; it is a process, and a largely cultural one, that bridges the diverse worlds of computing and medicine. Any health-care professional, or even patient, who has an idea for improving it or adding new applications can add the necessary code themselves, or pay a growing industry of VistA software consultants to do the work. And because these consultants are in competition with each other and have nothing to sell but their own skills and ingenuity, health-care providers (and, by extension, taxpayers and payers of health insurance premiums) won't have to pay them exorbitantly; the owners of proprietary software, on the other hand, know their customers can't easily go elsewhere if they want new features.

Most importantly, embracing VistA, and thwarting the further proliferation of proprietary health IT, advances science. Before science, there was alchemy, which went nowhere because alchemists didn't share their data and worked in secrecy. How can digital medicine be scientific if it is similarly based on a foundation of trade secrets and commercial rivalry? As one of the principle thought leacders behind open-source medicine, Dr. Ignacio Valdes has observed, "this is the choice that our nation faces, to become a nation of government certified health IT alchemy ushering in a medical digital dark age or a nation that reaffirms that transparency, and openness are the answer."[6]

TEN

Growing the VA

Gary Nickel, sixty-two, never liked to talk about his experiences in Vietnam. It's only recently that his wife, Terry, has gotten some details out of him about why he's started screaming in his sleep and locking his hands as if he is choking someone. He told her about the time when, at the giant Bien Hoa Air Base 20 miles northeast of Saigon, a plane landed and all the men jumped off puking. Nickels, whose job was to load and unload aircraft, discovered inside the rotting head of a U.S. soldier stuck on a post.

Gary told her, too, about his flashbacks to the many times during the Tet Offensive when he shook in bunkers while under mortar attack. After much objection about "not wanting to be pegged" with a mental illness, Gary at last relented to his wife's insistence that he seek treatment for post-traumatic stress syndrome and now takes pills prescribed by a private physician to treat it. But that's not his greatest medical need. Gary also suffers from Parkinson's disease, a degenerative disorder of the central nervous system that impairs motor and cognitive skills. Parkinson's is most often found among the elderly, but Gary was only fifty-six when he was first diagnosed, and he degenerated quickly.[1]

Within 2 years, Gary had to give up his job at the water treatment plant in Moorhead, Minnesota, and Terry had to give up her job as a nurse to stay with him around the clock. (The couple has no children.) Forced to live on a reduced income, including a $450-a-month Social Security disability check, they sold their home and bought a smaller, easier-to-navigate house furnished with a hospital bed, a trapeze, and special pillows to help with Gary's bedsores. Terry is also responsible these days for looking after her eighty-year-old mother, who now lives with them.

This might be just another sad story of another working-class American family struggling with poor luck and bad health, except that it gets worse in ways that involve us all. Terry thought it very important that she get her husband enrolled at the VA Medical Center in nearby Fargo, North Dakota, which would provide, among other benefits, equipment like the ramps he needs and, importantly, respite care for herself. She knew that, because of Gary's modest Social Security disability check, the couple wouldn't meet the VA's strict means test for admission. But she'd been reading about growing scientific evidence linking Parkinson's disease to exposure to Agent Orange—a chemical defoliant widely used in Vietnam. And as it happens, the Bien Hoa Air Base was and remains an Agent Orange hot spot in Vietnam, so much so that the U.S. government committed in 2008 to helping the Vietnamese government clean up the high levels of dioxins and other contaminants left behind.[2] So in 2007 Terry applied for Gary to be admitted to the VA, based on consideration of Parkinson's as a service-related illness.

The bureaucracy at the Fargo VA, however, was unmoved. Fourteen months after making their application, Gary and

Terry received a two-and-one-quarter page, single-spaced letter dated July 7, 2008, that spelled out the VA's rationale for rejecting Gary's enrollment. The case officer acknowledged finding a study on Wikipedia that showed that people exposed to herbicides like Agent Orange have "a 70 percent greater incidence of PD than individuals not exposed" but then went on to suggest that the real reason Gary contracted Parkinson's at such a young age could be "a 14-year history of smoking" or "occupational hazards" at the water plant. Terry says she assembled hundreds of pages of studies to rebut these claims—a tactic that has worked for a handful of Vietnam vets with Parkinson's. But after a year of waiting for the verdict on their appeal, she learned, with the help of local legislators, that the VA had simply closed their case. "In my eyes," Terry says softly, "it's all political."

Though she lost her battle, Terry turned out to be right on the facts. In the fall of 2009, the head of the VA, Eric K. Shinseki, acknowledged growing medical evidence linking Parkinson's and two other common diseases to Agent Orange. Yet Gary Nickels and hundreds of thousands of other vets have been made to suffer for years without care, thanks to a system that conditions benefits on scientific proof of a service-related disability—proof that accumulates so slowly that many veterans will be dead and buried before they're finally deemed eligible.

An essential step in health-care reform that is not only morally overdue but also highly practical is simply this: open up the VA. All veterans should have access to VA health-care benefits, with no questions asked about the ultimate (and often unknowable) causality of their illnesses.

Full access was once the law of the land. In signing the

Veterans' Health Care Eligibility Reform Act of 1996, President Clinton explained that it "authorizes the Department of Veterans Affairs to furnish comprehensive medical services to all veterans."[3] But then in 2003, under the Bush administration, the policy changed. The VA, having failed to receive the funding it needed to make good on the health care promised to millions of veterans, restricted new enrollments to those who either can meet a strict means test or have ailments directly and demonstrably related to military service. This is why Gary and Terry Nickel found themselves being chewed up by the VA's claims bureaucracy. It's also why, according to one recent study, there were fourteen times more vets under age sixty-five who died in 2008 due to lack of health insurance than there were soldiers killed fighting in Afghanistan.[4] And it is why, 10 or 20 years from now, many veterans of Afghanistan or Iraq will face ordeals similar to those faced by Nickels if they are forced to prove, for example, that they are afflicted by long-term complications from traumatic brain injuries (early onset dementia would not be a surprise). The better way forward, both for vets and for the country as a whole, is to open up the VA, even to the point of allowing family members of vets to buy into the system. Under that plan, which the major veterans service organizations endorse, the VA would become a model delivery system for a significant and diverse segment of the population, and it would point the way by example toward the creation of an equivalent, civilian institution.

The Lessons of Agent Orange

The ludicrousness of forcing vets, or anyone else, to prove that they are deserving of health care is underscored by the long and continuing struggle over Agent Orange, which offers a mirror to our society's confused thinking about the relationships among science, morality, and just desserts. You might well believe we took care of the Agent Orange problem years ago. Those of us beyond a certain age can remember the headlines, the angry demonstrations, the acrimonious hearings. We can remember how the government long denied that exposure to Agent Orange could contribute to any ill health save a case of chloracne—a disfiguring skin condition. How the gigantic class action suit against Dow, Monsanto, and other manufacturers of Agent Orange left Vietnam veterans furious over its miniscule out-of-court settlement. How Reagan's VA administrator, Robert Nimmo, used an appearance on NBC's *Today* show to call Vietnam veterans "a bunch of crybabies." How conservative think tanks denounced as "junk science" any studies implicating Agent Orange as a cause of illness. And how, finally, the federal government acknowledged the mounting scientific evidence linking Agent Orange to a variety of diseases and promised to make its victims whole.

On February 6, 1991, President George H.W. Bush signed the Agent Orange Act into law. It seemed like a great victory to Vietnam vets at the time. The legislation codified the provision that any Vietnam vet with any of three conditions known by then to be strongly associated with Agent Orange would automatically qualify for VA health care—no questions asked. And the bill called upon Institute of Medicine (IOM) to continuously look for new evidence of Agent Orange's long-term health-care effects. Backed by the great champion of veterans' causes, the late Democratic Congressman G.V. "Sonny" Montgomery, as well as by then Republican senator Arlen

Specter, the bill promised to bring closure to what Bush called "this very complex and very divisive issue."

For awhile, the legislation seemed to stand as an example of an overdue, but morally sound, workable policy based on science. In 1993, the IOM found a positive association between Agent Orange and Hodgkin's and several other comparatively rare diseases, and the VA dutifully added these to the list of conditions presumed to be service-connected for anyone who served in Vietnam. But as the years went by, the IOM and other researchers kept turning up more and more evidence of more and more complications from exposure to Agent Orange. A huge shocker, both to most Vietnam vets themselves and to federal budgeters, came in 2000 when the IOM reported a link between exposure to Agent Orange and type II diabetes—one of the most common diseases in America. It turns out to be substantially more common among Vietnam vets, and though it cost a bundle, the VA, under the waning Clinton administration, changed its rules so that all Vietnam vets with the condition are now presumed to have a service-related illness and therefore eligible for VA care.

Then, though it attracted little attention in a country that had moved on, the news kept getting worse. As Vietnam vets passed through their fifties and sixties, they turned out to be afflicted by high rates and early onsets of more and more chronic diseases, such as hypertension, and cancers of the lung and prostate, for which Agent Orange turned out to be a serious risk factor. Science also began confirming many suspicions about vets' children's health. In 2007, for example, the VA reported that 1,200 children of Vietnam veterans had spina bifida, a birth defect closely associated with a key ingredient of Agent Orange.

Then, in July of 2009, a bombshell landed on VA secretary Eric K. Shinseki's desk. In the most recent of a long series of reports titled *Veterans and Agent Orange*, the IOM added Parkinson's, ischemic heart disease, and hairy cell leukemia to its list of conditions associated with Agent Orange exposure, a list that has now grown to include, as well, hypertension, prostate cancer, cancer of the lung, and several more conditions.

In response, Shinseki ordered a rule change redefining Parkinson's, ischemic heart disease, and hairy cell leukemia as service-related illnesses for any Vietnam vet. Presuming those rules make it through final review, people like Gary Nickel and some 200,000 other vets will soon have a much easier time claiming benefits.

But what about vets who suffer from other conditions that have not yet been, but may someday be, linked to Agent Orange? For now, their only hope is to follow the route Gary Nickel took: try to prove the disease was caused by exposure to Agent Orange, to the satisfaction of some overwhelmed VA service officer who may well try to settle the matter with some scratching around on Wikipedia.

Dusted Off

Whether or not one's ill-health is related to military service or any other experience is usually a metaphysical question. By their very nature, almost all chronic disorders are multicausal, influenced by factors such as genetics, diet, behavior, and environmental influences, often all acting together. In Vietnam, the environment was saturated, not just with Agent Orange, but with a stew of other toxic chemicals whose effects could have been harmful in combination, though it would be extremely difficult to determine that scientifically. "Operation Flyswatter," for example, sprayed 1.76 million concentrated liters of the insecticide malathion over major bases and cities every 9 days as part of efforts to prevent malaria. Troops in the same areas were given "Monday pills," weekly doses of the antimalaria drug chloroquine, which turns out to inhibit an enzyme the body uses to help metabolize neurotoxins. "Bottom line," says Alan B. Oates, who heads the VA's Agent Orange committee, "Vietnam veterans were taking prescribed medication that reduced their body's ability to detoxify itself while being subjected to exposures of neurotoxins." (Personal communication)

There has been little study of how Agent Orange may have interacted with other toxins common in the environment of war-era Vietnam, which included DDT, paraquat, napalm, jet fuels, and many others. Further studies should be done. But we should also ask ourselves what, exactly, would we do with any new information? Yes, it is good to know all we can about the epidemiology of disease, but there are limits to what we can know, and dangers in using science inappropriately. Consider, for example, that even if all involved had acted in perfect good faith, science could not have discovered most of the long-term effects of Agent Orange and other toxic exposures except with the passage of time—time enough for Vietnam vets to start having large numbers of deformed children, and even more time for them to start developing Parkinson's in their fifties. And even then, all science can deliver are generalizations about large populations—not a determination of what caused any one person's chronic illness.

And so we have seen huge numbers of vets who have had

to endure the effects of Agent Orange without care or compensation until their own suffering and deaths at last produced enough scientific data to drive a change in policy. Normally, we want science to drive policy. But in this realm, waiting for science has meant waiting for an army to age and die, while also forcing sick veterans and their loved ones into the gears of a giant, overburdened, capricious claims bureaucracy—all for the purpose of trying to exclude the "undeserving."

Who is to say whether and how much Gary Nickel's career in water treatment plant contributed to Parkinson's, or what difference it should make in his access to government-provided health care? Today, it is harried, overworked—sometimes sympathetic, sometimes not—claims processors at the VA who make the call. Or it is the Board of Veterans' Appeals and the Court of Appeals for Veterans' Claims, which hear some 38,000 cases a year—a huge portion of them involving disputes over questions of causality and individual just desserts that ultimately have no scientific answers.

Back in the World

In retrospect, justice would have been far better served if we had just presumed all along that all Vietnam veterans deserved VA care, and it is still not too late to do that. Nor is it too late to do it for younger and older vets.

As a practical matter, the majority of our veterans are already old enough to qualify for Medicare, so taxpayers are on the hook for the cost of their care anyway. Does it make sense to exclude them from the VA when the VA delivers care at a lower cost per patient and enjoys higher patient satisfaction than Medicare?

The VA also has excess capacity in many parts of the country and will soon have much, much more as the once-giant ranks of World War II and Korean War vets grow thin. Meanwhile, the VA provides, for those who can get in, very high-quality care. We need to open up the VA and grow it. So long as the VA remains one of the, if not the, most cost-effective, scientifically driven, integrated health-care delivery systems in the country, the more patients it treats, the better for everyone.

Every vet should be able to use his or her insurance, including Medicare insurance, to receive treatment at the VA. Those who are indigent or who suffer from obvious war wounds should be given free care; others should contribute to the cost of their care as they are able. But any American who honorably served in the military should not find him- or herself locked out of the VA.

Then there's the effect on the taxpayers. One big, real-world consequence of the VA's current tight eligibility rules is a far bigger bill from Medicare. "I do not understand the logic," says Ken Kizer. He continues:

> The VA is providing more superior care, on a regular basis, than Medicare. Patient satisfaction is higher. You can show that it is doing it at a cost per patient of about half to two-thirds of Medicare. So why do you cut off people, tell them they can't go to the VA, and force them into Medicare? And why do you not allow Medicare patients to use their benefits at the VA? (Personal communication)

It's not as if such a step involves impossible politics. What conservative believes that our military isn't weakened when America breaks its promises to veterans? What health insurance industry lobbyist wants to be seen standing in the way of veterans getting needed health care? What liberal believes that showing solidarity with veterans and offering to restore health benefits cut under the Bush administration isn't politically shrewd? What taxpayer can't see the virtue of luring as many veterans as possible from Medicare and publicly subsidized insurance plans to lower-cost, higher-quality VA health care?

Family Medicine

The same logic leads to the next step on the road to comprehensive health reform. That step is to assure veterans, both young and old, that their spouses and dependant children can also join an expanding veterans' health-care system. Inclusion of families not only makes clinical sense—think of poor Terry Nickel's needs and the millions of aging veterans' wives like her—it also makes economic sense. It would allow, for example, an aging male veteran and his wife to be treated by a single primary care physician, who could deal with their codependencies and help them to manage each other's various chronic conditions.

Or take an example from the other end of life. Under current law, the VA may provide medical benefits to a woman during pregnancy and labor, but not to her baby. About a thousand female veterans a year are forced to seek care outside the VA system when their babies are due. How does this make sense?

In effect, the proposal here involves allowing military families to buy into the VA system while also giving those currently enrolled with Medicare or Medicaid the same option. Ken Kizer and others who have studied these options believe the VA could be financially self-sustaining if allowed to grow along these lines. The VA would become in effect an integrated, national network of nonprofit, staff-model HMOs and community clinics specializing in the treatment of military families. Once a year, veterans and their families would, through either their employer-sponsored plans or government-sponsored plans, have the option of electing for VA care, just as many today can decide whether to receive care through a Medicare Advantage Plan or a managed care network organized by their insurance network.

Could the VA handle a large increase in its patient load? Certainly, though not all at once. But remember, in cities and communities across America, dozens of veterans hospitals, as well as community hospitals, are slated for closure because they lack sufficient patients to maintain safe volumes of care. Remember, too, that the VA's twenty-first-century model of care does not require vast amounts of brick and mortar: its emphasis is on outpatient care, community clinics, and pre-vention of acute care needs, all making extensive use of infor-mation technology.

Bear in mind, also, the rapid decline in the numbers of vet-erans, which will soon free up much capacity. Currently at around 24 million, the veterans population will shrink to less than 19 million by 2019 and to 15.8 million by 2029. Even with all the men and women who have served in Afghanistan and Iraq, the number of active-duty U.S military personnel as of 2006 was only about a third of what it was in the 1980s, and only a tenth of what it was in 1945.

The drop-off in the numbers of very old veterans, who tend to place the most demand on veterans hospitals, will be par-ticularly sharp over the next 20 years. The number of veterans eighty-five and over, for example, is expected to decline from 253,385 in 2006 to 162,032 in 2026. After that, the number of very old veterans will begin to rise again, as Vietnam vets age into their eighties and beyond. But through at least 2033 there will not be as many veterans eighty-five or over as today—a trend exactly opposite the trend in the aging U.S. population as a whole.[5]

So why are we making it increasingly harder for veterans to get access to the veterans' health-care system? For far too many sick veterans, especially those who served in Vietnam, experiencing a rejection like Gary Nickel endured is taken as the final insult of an ungrateful nation. It's a hard way to die. For the rest of us, joining their cause not only is morally right, but also advances the mission of true health reform by bringing us closer to establishing the principle that access to affordable quality health care should not have to be earned but is a right of citizenship.

ELEVEN

....

The Vista Life Network

Back in July 2007, while trying to justify his opposition to expanding government health-care coverage for children, President Bush made a telling comment. The uninsured, he said, "have access to health care in America. After all, you just go to an emergency room."[1]

That remark struck many as blithe and callous, and it was. The uninsured don't receive in ERs anything like the health care they need. Indeed, lack of insurance increases mortality by 44 percent, according to a recent study by the Harvard School of Public Health and the Cambridge Health Alliance.[2] Just try getting a dose of chemotherapy or dialysis by going to the ER.

Still, there was a kernel of truth to Bush's comment—one that we ought to take as a jumping-off point for rethinking how to reform the health-care system beyond the VA. The nation has long had an extensive, if ad hoc, system for providing health care to the uninsured. Some of that care is delivered at the suburban hospitals and doctors' offices where those of us with health insurance generally get treated. But the lion's share of health care for the uninsured has long been provided by assorted "St. Elsewhere" institutions—typically big, old,

nonprofit community or teaching hospitals in poorer neighborhoods—with additional help from smaller public clinics.

A fair amount of money flows through that system.
Americans who lacked health insurance in 2004 received an
average of $1,629 per person in medical services, which is
more than the total average per capita health-care expenditure in Europe.³ More surprisingly, the quality of care they
received is, by some important measures, *better* than that of
insured Americans.

Insured Against Overtreatment

Yes, that's right. A landmark RAND study, published in
the *New England Journal of Medicine*, has found for example
that uninsured patients receive only 53.7 percent of the
care experts believe they should get, which is a tragedy. But
according to the same study, patients with private, fee-for-
service insurance are even less likely to receive appropriate,
evidence-based treatment. Indeed, among Americans receiving acute care, those who lack insurance stand a slightly
better chance of receiving proper treatment than patients
covered by Medicaid, Medicare, or any form of private
insurance.⁴

How can this be, you might ask? Turns out that being
uninsured paradoxically provides insurance against some of
the leading causes of death and injury in the United States.
Overtreatment, for example. Once patients who are unable to
pay are in a hospital's door, they cost it money until its doctors
make them well enough to leave. There is no incentive what-
soever to give them tests or treatments they don't need. Since
about 30 percent of all health-care spending in the United

States goes for overtreatment—much of it dangerous—this no small advantage.

Also, the less time you spend in a hospital, the less likely you are to contract a staph infection, or to be killed or maimed by medical errors. Similarly, not having health insurance tends to reduce your exposure to ionizing radiation from imaging devices. With the possible exception of mammography, these scans provide no proven benefits yet are a growing cause of cancer, particularly among persons who have received repeated radiation exposures—typically well-insured elderly patients.[5] As a recent commentary in the *New England Journal of Medicine* observed, "Exposure to even moderate degrees of medical radiation presents an important yet potentially avoidable public health threat"—one that the uninsured by and large do not have to worry about.[6]

You might think that at least insured Americans get better preventive care, what with their $10 copays to see a physician. Also not true. According to the RAND study, patients with private fee-for-service insurance receive only 53.3 percent of the preventive care they need, while those *without* insurance receive 54 percent.[7] Even HMOs, though they do slightly better on this score, face the reality that their patients are constantly churning from one plan to the next and so, as we've seen, don't have a business case for investment in true prevention. Meanwhile, fee-for-service providers will happily charge you for a high-radiation, full-body, three-dimensional, sixty-four-slice (cancer-causing) scan of no proven diagnostic value, and call it prevention.

Harvard biochemist Lawrence J. Henderson, one of the Progressive Era's most renowned men of science, once observed that it wasn't until somewhere around 1911 that the progress of medicine at last made it possible to say that "a random patient with a random disease consulting a physician at random stood better than a 50-50 chance of benefiting from the encounter."[8] Sadly, the RAND data and a growing pile of other studies suggest that this statement is essentially still true today, for those with or without insurance.

It's also true, as we've seen, that the nation's public hospitals, while they may have a Dickensian atmosphere and lack valet parking, tend to deliver higher-quality health care than their more prestigious counterparts. Whether suffering from heart attacks, colon cancer, or hip fractures, patients live longer if they stay away from "elite" hospitals, with their overabundance of specialists, and choose a lower-cost St. Elsewhere. Given this unexpected reality, it is perhaps not surprising that patient satisfaction also declines as a hospital's spending per patient rises. It's not fun to be overtested and overtreated, even if you're fully insured and get valet parking and the finest in pudding.[9]

This focus on overtreatment is not to minimize the plight of the uninsured. Aggregate statistics mask huge suffering and disparities in treatment, particularly for painful, chronic conditions. But the fact that uninsured patients are more likely to receive quality acute care and preventive care than do those with insurance ought to make us question what real health reform would look like. For years, the debate over health care has rested on the assumption that the uninsured should be brought into the health-care system the rest of us use. But what if something like the opposite is true? What if the best way to help the uninsured is to make the health-care delivery system they already use—the St. Elsewhere model—better, more efficient, and more affordable—in short, more like the VA? And what if, eventually, the rest of us could join that system?

The Vista Health Care Network

What I'm proposing is this: Take the existing ad hoc system we've been using for treating the uninsured, and turn it into a real integrated system. Specifically, insure the uninsured by whatever means. But then, don't just wait for the inevitable increase in demand to swamp an already sinking system. Take the next essential, logical step—and quickly: recruit assorted St. Elsewheres and individual doctors to become part of an integrated health-care delivery system serving the vastly expanded pool of newly insured patients, and make the organizing blueprint of this new system the one successful, fully integrated, national health-care system we currently have: the VA.

For purposes of discussion, let's imagine that this new civilian VA took the name Vista Health Care Network, because it had been inspired by the VA's best-in-class VistA electronic medical record system and the high-quality model of care that the system makes possible. The slogan for the Vista Heath Care Network could be "Health for Life"—because Vista's prime long-term objective would be to offer Americans continuous and integrated lifetime care similar to that enjoyed by patients in the VA system.

Some wonkish readers steeped in the jargon of today's emerging debate over system delivery reform might say: "Oh, you mean set up an accountable care organization and pay its doctors fee for value instead of fee for service, using a comparative effectiveness board to set protocols." Yes, that is close to what I am saying, but with the important added message that we don't need, and don't have time for, endless studies and pilot programs to show how it could be done. With only a few tweaks, the VA provides us with a proven model because it was an "accountable care organization" long before most health-care wonks had any such concept.

The first task of the Vista network's board would be to approach various public and charitable hospitals around the country and offer them a deal: Let us help you install the VA's VistA health information management software, and agree to adhere to the performance measures and protocols of evidence-based medicine used by the VA itself. In exchange, you will get a contract to care for a guaranteed pool of people— who will be paid for.

Initially, these would be people who cannot afford, without subsidy, to comply with an individual mandate requiring all Americans to acquire health insurance. They might include people covered by Medicaid, a public option insurance plan, a co-op, a private carrier participating in a "public exchange"— whatever. Such people could opt for any provider network included in these insurance plans, but the default setting would be for care provided by the Vista Health Care Network. Reimbursement rates would be set much higher than in Medicaid, and when combined with the efficiency in the VA model of care, they'd be high enough to guarantee the solvency of participating providers.

It wouldn't be hard for the Vista board to find hospitals willing to take this deal. Across the country, community hospitals are going bankrupt. Moreover, one of the likely effects of the current round of health insurance reform will be dramatic cuts in Medicaid and Medicare reimbursement rates for big, urban St. Elsewheres that don't improve their efficiency. Let's put ourselves in the shoes of people who manage, work for, or depend on one of these financially imperiled institutions.

Joining the Vista network would offer a lifeline. Yes, the hospitals that take Vista's offer would have to radically change the way they do business. They'd have to join the twenty-first century and integrate health IT into the practice of medicine. They'd have to embrace the VA's safety culture. They'd also have to shed acute care beds and specialists and invest in more outpatient clinics in which, for example, diabetics could learn how to manage their disease, or people with high blood pressure could join smoking-cessation and exercise programs. As with the VA, there would also be much more emphasis on integrated mental health–care and substance-abuse programs.

Also as with the VA, doctors who work for these hospitals would be salaried and earn bonuses for effective performance (keeping their patients well). No longer would doctors have a financial incentive to engage in overtreatment. Nor would they be constantly visited by gift-bearing pill "detailers," because decisions on what prescription drugs to use would be made on a scientific basis by the institution as a whole and because the Vista network, like the VA, would negotiate as an institution to obtain the best prices from drug companies.

Importantly, however, the cost savings that Vista would achieve would not come primarily from jawboning on the price it paid for drugs, medical devices, lab tests, etc., as could well be true of a plan that simply offered a public option for health-care insurance. As Princeton health economist Uwe Reinhardt has pointed out, a public option for health insurance could, by increasing competition among insurance companies, have the unintended effect of reducing their market power in negotiating for lower-cost drugs and reimbursement rates. This reduced power would leave participants in the public plan better off, but everyone else worse off.[10] In contrast, the Vista system would achieve most of its cost savings, not by pushing costs off onto others, but by adhering to a model of care that is inherently more efficient due to its effective use of health IT, evidence-based medicine, and all the other factors already discussed. Other health-care providers could effectively compete with Vista so long as they adopted an equally or more efficient model of health care, which is the form of competition we want in health care.

Though Vista would ruffle many feathers, it would make winners out of many institutions that would otherwise be losers. Accepting the Vista deal means that many currently imperiled hospitals wouldn't have to close. Instead, the local community could take pride in having preserved an institution that not only serves the needy, but offers them high-quality, high-value health care as well. As long as the hospital and its clinics demonstrably adhered to the VA's evidence-based model of care, local politicians could continue to use it as a source of patronage, while local restaurants, stores, and real estate agents could continue to live off the income its employees spread throughout the community.

Beyond money-starved St. Elsewheres, the few other health-care providers who are already practicing medicine on a model approximating that of the VA might be tempted to join the Vista system. For institutions such as Kaiser Permanente and Intermountain Healthcare, for example, joining the Vista network, or forming a division that does, would not require great changes in their cultures and day-to-day operation, because they already, in comparison to other non-VA providers, make effective use of health IT and evidence-based medicine. Joining Vista could help them to expand into new markets and geographical areas they currently are having trouble penetrating because of the lack of an effective business case for quality in medicine outside of the VA. Participation in Vista would offer such institutions something approximating the VA's lifelong relationship with its patients, and also a funding mechanism that rewarded quality. Also, such institutions would gain the considerable sales point that enrollees, wherever they might happen to be when they got sick, could receive coordinated treatment from an integrated national network of Vista-affiliated providers. Participation in Vista would also help such institutions achieve further economies of scale in technology, purchasing, information management, and marketing.

Now, let's put ourselves in the shoes of those who would be the customers of the new Vista system. One segment would be people with lower incomes, who for the most part are already frequenting the ERs of various St. Elsewheres for their health-care needs. For those customers, the transition to the new, integrated, rationalized system would be easy and welcome. They would be able to get preventive care, such as regular doctor checkups, as well as chronic care, such as effective management of diabetes, and not face the stigma and stress of medical bankruptcy.

A second segment of Vista customers would be mostly young people. Many of them might not like being forced to buy insurance, because they might think they don't need it. But if they were required to, they'd likely see the Vista network as an attractive option because of its low cost and its nationwide presence, which would mean they wouldn't have to change health-care plans when they move. Younger people, too, are more likely than their parents and grandparents to recognize the benefits of electronic medical records and the evidence-based care they make possible.

For all this to work, Vista would need to have what the VA already enjoys: a lifetime relationship with the bulk of its patients so that its financial incentives would be in line with its patients' health needs. Such a relationship could happen with a relatively modest legal fix: anyone in the Vista system who got a job that offered health insurance should be allowed to direct his or her employer to pay premiums to the Vista system if he or she wanted to remain in the system. Elders would also be allowed to use their Medicare coverage to enroll with Vista, which, if the VA's performance is matched, would both increase the quality of care and save taxpayer dollars. And, presuming the system worked well, most people would want to stay in it, given its national reach and most people's strong desire not to have to constantly change doctors and health plans.

Not all, but many, doctors are likely to welcome the program. Those joining the Vista system would be free of the hassle of having to file claims to third-party payers and, as in the case of VA doctors, would not bear the burden of paying for medical malpractice insurance. Idealistic doctors and other health-care professionals would be particularly attracted to the network, as they are to the VA, because it would allow them to pursue best practices in medicine without being compromised by the dictates of profit-maximizing insurance companies and hospital shareholders. Again as with the VA, Vista doctors would be a self-selected group of medical professionals who would not be "in it for the money," which is just what we want. Help with paying down medical school debt could be a further recruiting tool if it turned out to be needed.

Creating a Vista Health Care Network would not require the government to incur huge capital costs or long-term debt. Though the network might have to build some of its own hospitals and clinics in certain underserved locations, most Vista-affiliated facilities would remain owned and operated by the private interests, charity organizations, and local governments that currently run them. Use of a common IT platform (VistA) would allow for system-wide monitoring of individual hospital, clinic, and doctor performance while also allowing for the data mining needed to advance outcomes research and refine evidence-based protocols of care.

By building on a system that already exists, then, the Vista plan would be the least costly and, initially, the least disruptive way to provide the uninsured with health care (and high-quality care, at that). But this doesn't mean health-care lobbyists wouldn't go after Vista. They would. For while Vista would not, in the short run, pose a large challenge to the private-sector health-care market, in the long run it would be a different story.

Again, the VA experience is instructive. Thanks to quality improvements, many veterans not currently eligible for VA health-care benefits are demanding access to VA hospitals. Similarly, imagine that Vista were put into place and worked as advertised. Over time, word would get out that the quality of treatment in Vista was pretty good—indeed, better than what most people with employer-provided health care receive. Pretty soon, individuals who were not eligible for Vista would start clamoring for the right to buy into the system. And employers, realizing that Vista was doing a better job of controlling costs than their own private-sector health providers, would start pressuring Washington for permission to contract with Vista to provide health care for their employees.

If this kind of competition were allowed to happen, private health-care companies would either lose customers to Vista or be forced to find ways to curb overtreatment, reduce medical errors, and in general provide better, more cost-efficient care. Either way, the competition would lead to dramatic improvements in American health care. Just as the existence of state universities puts competitive pressure on private universities to pursue excellence, the existence of the Vista network, a true public option, would force the rest of the health-care system to try matching it on quality and value.

Blowback

Is this proposal politically feasible? Importantly, the Vista plan offers a hands-on, credible strategy for controlling costs while improving quality. This is key to attracting the support of the majority of Americans, who are rightfully concerned about adding new, open-ended entitlements to the country's welfare state at a time of mounting debts. They remember how health-care costs exploded beyond all predictions after the introduction of Medicare. They now hear how Medicare, while covering only a fraction of the population, has wracked up $38 trillion in unfunded liabilities and is expected to exhaust its trust fund in a few short years. They hear bold talk about "pilot programs" in Medicare to rein in spending and improve quality, but they see no reason why "Medicare for everyone" wouldn't make the country go broke just that much quicker. By taking on the delivery system directly, using a proven model, the Vista plan would have more potential political appeal than any single-payer proposal, even while it drew fire from doctors and hospitals who currently profit from wasteful spending.

Today's progressives should not forget that back in the 1960s, Wilbur J. Cohen and the other original architects of Medicare thought they where establishing a "beachhead" for universal health-care insurance. They figured that once younger Americans saw how well Medicare worked for the elderly, there would be a demand that Medicare be expanded to cover all ages. Yet largely because the then overwhelming power of the American Medical Association forced the architects of Medicare to focus exclusively on expanding coverage, as opposed to reforming the actual delivery of health care, Medicare's costs exploded. And those exploding costs became the chief political reason why the cause of universal coverage stalled for two generations, as even many liberals came to think of it as simply unaffordable.

Any major health insurance reform could well backfire again if it is not joined to something like the Vista network. Without it, most Americans would see their premiums continuing to rise while they experienced more crowded waiting rooms and a continuing breakdown in day-to-day medical practice. Such an experience would inevitably reinforce the idea in yet another generation of Americans that government involvement in health care is categorically a bad idea, despite all the contrary evidence available from the VA and from national health-care systems around the world.[11]

A plan like Vista could help avoid backlash in other ways

as well. Its comparative "thriftiness" could make it appealing to fiscal conservatives. Also, while it would, to be sure, expand the role of government in the direct provision of health care, no one would be compelled by law to join the Vista network, just as no one is compelled to receive treatment at the VA. In replicating the best features of the VA, Vista might offer the best care anywhere, but its existence would not erode our all-American right to make bad choices in health care.

Importantly, too, the model for Vista comes, not from Canada or France, but from an all-American institution widely cheered by the nation's veterans. If the system is good enough for our wounded warriors who have risked their lives for our country, how is it not good enough for civilians receiving publicly subsidized health insurance? Moreover, we don't have to guess how the VA model of care works or to decide the question on ideological grounds. We can just ask friends, neighbors, or relatives who use the system, or listen to what their advocates, such as the American Legion, have to say. They are bound to point out flaws but also to add that they get better care at the VA than elsewhere.

Moreover, framed correctly, this proposal for government provision of health care, as opposed to government provision of mere health insurance, should not seem out of step with American tradition. After all, American governments don't insure people against fire; instead they operate fire departments. American governments don't provide education insurance, but rather public schools. Nor do American governments underwrite auto insurance; instead they build roads and highways. Similarly, American governments don't offer flight insurance; they build airports and traffic control systems. Nor do we try to hedge against the risk of violence with an insurance plan; instead, governments organize police and military power to provide for collective security. None of this is considered socialism. How is government-provided health care fundamentally different?

Also, it is important to note that if this proposal does, for the time being, prove to be politically unfeasible on a national scale, any state has the opportunity to initiate its own Vista health network, or something like it. This would be a great way for states to contain their exploding Medicaid costs, for example. It could even be done regionally or by individual cities if they were allowed the necessary waivers to state and federal laws. To the extent that this model of care drove down health-care cost while enhancing quality and patient satisfaction, it would provide a comparative advantage to locations at any level in attracting new industry and holding on to existing jobs.

Yes, there is a solution to the health-care crisis. It starts with the comparatively limited step of creating a high-quality, cost-effective, health-care delivery system available to all veterans and to the 47 million Americans and counting who cannot afford private health insurance without subsidy. It ends with all Americans wondering why we took so long to open our hearts and our minds and create a Vista "Health for Life" network available to everyone.

Epilogue

On January 15, 2006, the City of New York began requiring local clinical laboratories to report the results of blood sugar tests performed on individual citizens to the city's health department. The department plans to use the information to improve surveillance for diabetes, which now afflicts an estimated one out of eight New Yorkers, and to "target interventions." Specifically, if you live in New York and have trouble resisting sweets or exercising regularly, your doctor may well soon receive a call from the health department suggesting the need to persuade you to change your lifestyle.

What makes this development so extraordinary in the annals of American public health is that diabetes is not a disease you can catch from, or give to, anyone else. To be sure, American governments have a long history of imposing quarantines and otherwise restricting the liberties of people suspected of carrying contagious disease. Early in the last century, for example, the very same New York City Health Department famously exiled Mary Mallon (a.k.a. "Typhoid Mary"), along with many other infectious patients, to a tiny island "colony" in the East River.

Existing policies requiring the reporting of sexually transmitted diseases to public health authorities similarly derive justification from the threat of contagion. Even recently enacted smoking bans in New York City and elsewhere only passed after the public accepted findings that "secondhand" smoke poses a serious health threat to others.

But diabetes, though now a fearsome epidemic, is not communicable; nor do the behaviors that lead to or exacerbate the disease (primarily lack of exercise and improper diet) put others at risk of illness. It cannot even be said of diabetics, as is often said of illegal drug users, that their habits foster a life of crime or fund crime syndicates and terrorist networks. So how does it become a matter of public interest that the governments surveil the medical records of individual citizens for telltale signs of high blood sugar, much less "target interventions"? Isn't this the ultimate example of the "nanny state" run amok?

Many readers may have similar fears about the implications of government-controlled electronic medical records and the VA model of health care that these records enable. Many people like the fact that they can consult doctors without them necessarily knowing that they once checked themselves into a psychiatric clinic, or sought treatment for alcoholism or drug abuse, or once had an abortion or venereal disease. Many people also don't want their doctors, let alone an agency of the government, haranguing them about their lifestyle—whether it be smoking, lack of exercise, eating sweets or fats, or whatever—any more than we want our auto mechanics telling us how to drive. Still others fear that their electronic medical records will fall into the wrong hands, thereby subjecting them to blackmail, identity theft, or discrimination by employers and insurance companies.

These are all understandable fears. Some can be allayed by technology. VistA is constructed so that researchers who mine the data contained in medical records cannot know whose records they are. Moreover, stealing electronic medical records without detection is often more difficult than stealing paper records. A paper record, for example, shows no sign if it has been photocopied, but VistA keeps a log of everyone who accesses the system and what they do within it.

Yet no one should pretend that a system like VistA does not pose threats to privacy. In 2006, the VA endured justified criticism when a laptop containing individual medical records was stolen from an employee's home.

The question is, are these threats sufficient to negate all the proven advantages VistA brings to the practice of medicine?

A hard truth is emerging in our time that should caution against snap judgments about the sanctity of medical privacy above all other values and goals in health care. Certainly we should continue to expect that our health-care records, both paper and electronic, be protected against theft and unauthorized access, and to demand that institutions that are sloppy about their responsibility to protect our records be punished. But maintaining medical privacy in any broader sense is becoming increasingly expensive, both to individuals and to the public. The emerging question is whether medical privacy is simply a basic human right or something more akin to a privilege for which those who want it should pay rather than shifting the cost onto others.

The primary reason for the increasing cost of medical privacy is the increasing prevalence of chronic diseases like diabetes. Such diseases, which have now become the leading causes of illness and death in advanced societies, typically cannot be prevented, cured, nor even much ameliorated, except by changes in diet and lifestyle that most of us, including myself, are disinclined, perhaps even genetically, to make. The Centers for Disease Control and Prevention attribute nearly half of all deaths in the United States to lifestyle causes, including alcohol consumption (3.5 percent of all deaths) obesity and poor nutrition (16.5 percent), and smoking (18 percent).[1]

The medical treatment of chronic diseases also typically requires highly coordinated and continuous care. It usually involves an array of specialists engaged in care ranging from surgery to intensive patient education, physical therapy, attempted behavioral modification, and, especially in the case of diabetes, constant monitoring. The coordination of such treatment requires sharing of patient information among a broad range of medical professionals, both at any given time and over time. Today, one in seven hospital admissions occurs because care providers do not have access to previous medical records. One out of five lab tests are done for the same reason.[2]

Moreover, advancing our understanding of how best to cure and manage such diseases requires assembling vast amounts of medical data about populations as a whole. There can be no "evidence-based" medicine without collecting evidence about what actually works for most people most of the time. Lack of free-flowing information in the health-care system drives up the cost of health insurance and contributes to the problem of the uninsured. For the population as a whole, it impedes the safe and effective practice of medicine, retards the development of medical protocols based on science, and in all these ways and more reduces productivity and life expectancy.

These are among the big reasons why a broad consensus has emerged, ranging from Hillary Clinton to Newt Gingrich, behind the idea that every American should have a lifelong electronic medical record. But the tradeoff to any increase in the flow of medical information is of course a threat to individual privacy. Deciding in what circumstances the tradeoffs are worth it is the new threshold issue in American health care. Medical privacy is not simply a question of individual right, even for individuals whose medical problems might at first seem purely their own concern.

The creation of a Vista Health system would remove, or at least seriously diminish, one major concern people have about their medical privacy. Enrollment in the system would be open to all, regardless of preexisting conditions. No one would ever again face the prospect of being unable to get health insurance, or to get it at a reasonable price, just because they once tested positive for AIDS or had a cancer tumor detected.

At the same time, however, Vista Health would probably take much more interest in your personal behavior than do the doctors you currently see. Following the VA's clinical guidelines, VA doctors routinely grill their patients about their smoking habits, for example. A survey of VA patients who smoke found that two-thirds had been counseled to quit by their doctor at least once within the last year.[3] Because of its long-term relationship with its patients, the VA has a strong institutional interest in deterring even its youngest patients from unhealthy habits. The VA estimates that smoking, for example, accounts for up to 24 percent of its total health-care costs—an expense that is driven up in large measure by the fact that the VA's smokers typically don't move on to other health-care plans before they begin experiencing smoking-related illnesses. Accordingly, the VA not only includes counseling against smoking in its clinical guidelines but charges no copayments for smoking cessation programs, associated drugs, or nicotine patches, the dollar cost of which, for most "civilian" smokers, matches or exceeds that of smoking itself.[4] The Vista Health system, facing the same institutional incentives to promote wellness, would show the same concern—or "nosiness" if that's how you regard it—about your lifestyle and long-term health.

Could such nosiness eventually be taken so far that it became a serious affront to personal liberty? Sure it could. In my view, the war on drugs is an egregious example of government excess committed in the name of preserving the population's health. But the point remains that medical privacy, far from being free, is getting more expensive all the time, due mostly to the changing nature of disease, which is more and more the result of behavioral and environmental factors. The true libertarian therefore asks, why should I pay for your privacy?

Enacting Vista Health does not mean that every American has to have a lifetime electronic health record or be treated by a system that has institutional incentives to promote wellness. Nor does it mean that individuals would have to give up their current doctors or forfeit the ability to pick out a new doctor in the future. Those who object to Vista's model of care on whatever grounds would still have the option of going to other sources.

They might thereby find themselves subjected to unnecessary surgeries, high risk of medical errors, and neglect of prevention, as well as being enabled in their addictions and bad habits. Or they might even have the rare but happy experience of finding that one specialist who provides a treatment that, though it's ineffective or harmful to most people, nonetheless works for them.

But choosing to opt out of the Vista Health system would probably cost you a lot of money. Private insurers would likely be glad to sell you a policy that covers care outside the Vista network, including care that is fragmented and unmanaged and that still clings to nineteenth-century information technology. But the premiums you would have to pay for such a policy would likely be very much higher than those charged by Vista Health.

One reason is the care you would be receiving would be inherently less efficient, more dangerous, less effective, and therefore more costly. Another reason is that your private health-care insurer would have to charge you a large "risk premium" to overcome the problem of adverse selection. The underwriters would be forced to consider that you have opted out of lower-cost Vista Health because you are looking for heroic or unproven treatments not offered by Vista—a risk to their capital for which they will have to charge you.

Also, the more medical information you insist remain unknown to the insurance company, such as the results of lab tests, the higher the premium the underwriters will have to charge you to overcome the uncertainty created by your demand for privacy. Any asymmetry of information between insurer and insuree necessarily drives up the cost of insurance. In a coming age of effective genetic testing and other means of better predicting individual susceptibility to disease, the price of medical privacy may well rise so high as to wreck the private health insurance market for all but the super rich or super fit.[5]

This, I believe, is the future of twenty-first-century medicine. One tendency of modern society is for us to become convinced of our individuality. We increasingly come to see ourselves as unique, not only in how our minds work but also our bodies. At the same time, we come to see ourselves as endowed with a bundle of universal liberties, including the freedom to eat, drink, or smoke whatever, drive wherever, sleep with whomever, and then choose whichever doctors and medical treatments we might want to try to deal with the consequences.

Yet a countervailing tendency heightens our objective dependency on others, however much we may hate to admit it. The percentage of the population suffering with chronic health conditions increases year after year. The percentage of Americans who can pay for their own health care decreases year after year. Progress in medicine continues, but as new drugs and treatment options proliferate, the consumer becomes lost in a sea of competing claims. Can Lexapro really cure generalized anxiety disorder? Does the syndrome really exist, and how could I tell if I had it? How can I tell if arthroscopic knee surgery is right for me, let alone find a surgical team that can perform the operation without giving me a staph infection? Such questions cannot be answered with a Google search.

Reconciling these two tendencies—increased individualism combined with increased objective dependence on others—will be a central theme of American politics for years to come. Neither pure socialized medicine nor pure market-driven medicine offers an acceptable solution. But giving all Americans the option to try out the high-quality, cost-effective model of care pioneered by the VA will make for a stronger and healthier nation while also preserving our individual right as Americans to make the wrong decision.

Acknowledgments

I am grateful to the many people who agreed to lend their time, expertise, and support as I set out to find a model for health-care delivery-system reform and absorb its paradoxical lessons. I am particularly indebted to Dr. Donald Berwick of the Institute for Health Care Improvement and Dr. Elliott S. Fisher of Dartmouth Medical School for teaching me new ways to look at health care. Dr. Kenneth Dickie, formerly of the VA, not only sat with me for an extensive interview but also provided me with invaluable access to his personal archive of material related to the VA's early and tumultuous experiments with digitalized health care. Dr. Scott Shreeve, founder of Medsphere—a company committed to bringing the VA model of care to the private sector—was also very generous with his time, insights, and archives, as has been Dr. Ken Kizer, who is now Medsphere's chair.

My colleague Shannon Brownlee and I have deeply influenced each other's thinking on health care over the years as we reported on—and tried to make sense of—the actual practice patterns of American medicine. For those interested in a deeper look at what's wrong with American medicine outside the VA, I recommend her book, *Overtreated: Why Too Much Medicine Is Making Us Sicker and Poorer* (Bloomsbury 2007).

Thanks go as well to Paul Glastris, editor in chief of the *Washington Monthly*, for his help in formulating many of the ideas in this book and for having the courage to publish my 2005 cover story on the VA. Len Nichols and Sherle Schwenninger of the New America Foundation provided useful comments and challenges. Brian Beutler provided invaluable research help, and Jeannette Warren provided essential editing of the early manuscripts. Deep thanks go to Bernard L. Schwartz, whose generous support of the foundation provided me with the time and intellectual freedom I needed to research and write this book. I also thank Peter Richardson and Scott Jordan of PoliPoint Press for their faith in this project and encouragement to produce a second edition. Finally, I am most grateful to my wife, Sandy, without whose thoughts, encouragement, and forbearance I could not have completed this book.

Notes

Preface to the Second Edition

1. Zhang J. The digital pioneer. *Wall Street Journal*, October 27, 2009. http://online.wsj.com/article/SB1000142405297020448830457442875013 3812262.html?mod=wsj_share_linkedin#printMode.

2. Congressional Budget Office. The health care system for veterans: an interim report. December 2007. http://www.cbo.gov/ftpdocs/88xx/doc8892/Frontmatter.1.3.shtml.

3. Cannon MF. VHA is not the way. nationalreview.com, March 6, 2006. http://www.cato.org/pub_display.php?pub_id=5847.

4. Starfield B. Is U.S. health really the best in the world? *Journal of the American Medical Association* 2000; 284(4):483–485.

5. Committee on the Consequences of Uninsurance, Institute of Medicine. *Care Without Coverage: Too Little, Too Late.* Washington, DC: National Academies Press; 2002; Wilper AP, Woolhandler S, Lasser KE, McCormick D, Bor DH, Himmelstein DU. Health insurance and mortality in U.S. adults. *American Journal of Public Health,* December 2009, vol. 99, no. 12.

6. New England Healthcare Institute. Waste and inefficiency in the U.S. healthcare system— clinical care: a comprehensive analysis in support of system-wide improvements. February 2008; Mahar M. The state of the nation's health. *Dartmouth Medicine,* Spring 2007; Kelley R. Where can $700 billion in waste be cut annually from the U.S. healthcare system? Thomson Reuters, October 2009.

Introduction

1. Corrigan J, et al, eds. *To Err Is Human: Building a Safer Health System.* Washington, DC: Institute of Medicine, the National Academies Press;

2000; editorial, Preventing fatal medical errors, *New York Times,* December 1, 1999, p. 22a.

2. Himmelstein DU, et al. Illness and injury as contributors to bankruptcy. *Health Affairs* (Millwood) 2005; Jan–Jun; Suppl Web Exclusives:W5-63–W5-73. http://www.healthaffairs.org/ (Type name of article in Web site's search box.) http://content.healthaffairs.org/cgi/search?ck=nck&andorexactfulltext=and&resourcetype=1&disp_type=&fulltext=Himmelstein+Illness+and+injury+as+contributors+to+bankruptcy+2005.

3. Chernew M, Hirth RA, Cutler DM. Increased spending on health care: long-term implications for the nation, *Health Affairs,* September/October 2009; 28(5): 1253–1255.

4. Cox M, Alm R. Time well spent: the declining real cost of living in America. 1997 Annual Report, Federal Reserve Bank of Dallas.

5. Blendon RJ, Benson JM. Americans' views on health policy: a fifty-year historical perspective. *Health Affairs* 2001; 20(2):39, Exhibit 5.

6. National Center for Health Statistics. *Health, United States, 2008, with Chartbook on Trends in the Health of Americans.* Hyattsville, MD: NCHS; 2009, Table 26. Life expectancy at birth, at 65 years of age, and at 75 years of age.

7. Bunker JP. The role of medical care in contributing to health improvements within societies. *International Journal of Epidemiology* 2001; 30:1260–1263. http://ije.oxfordjournals.org/cgi/content/full/30/6/1260.

8. Cutler DM, et al. The value of medical spending in the United States, 1960–2000. *New England Journal of Medicine* 2006; 355(9):920–927. http://content.nejm.org/cgi/content/full/355/9/920#R11. Numbers are adjusted to present value.

9. Strunk BC, Ginsburg PB. Aging plays limited role in health care cost trends. Center for the Study of Health System Change, Data Bulletin no. 23, September 2002, http://www.hschange.com/CONTENT/473/.

10. Boden WE, O'Rourke RA, Teo KK, Hartigan PM, Maron DJ, Kostuk WJ, et al. Optimal medical therapy with or without PCI for stable coronary disease. *New England Journal of Medicine.* 2007:26; 356(15):1503–16. Cecil WT, et al, A meta-analysis update: percutaneous coronary interventions. *American Journal of Managed Care.* 2008; 14(8):521–528.

11. Deyo RA. Back surgery—who needs it? *New England Journal of Medicine* 2007; 356: 2239–2243.

12. For a useful summary of this sad chapter in American medicine, see Welch HG, Mogielnicki J. Presumed benefit: lessons from the American experience with marrow transplantation for breast cancer. *British Medical Journal* 2002; 324:1088–1092.

13. Fisher ES, Bynum JP, Skinner JS. Slowing the growth of health care costs—lessons from regional variation. *New England Journal of Medicine* 2009; 360:849–852. http://content.nejm.org/cgi/content/full/360/9/849

14. Waste and inefficiency in the U.S. healthcare system—clinical care: a comprehensive analysis in support of system-wide improvements. New England Healthcare Institute, February 2008; Mahar M. The state of the nation's health. *Dartmouth Medicine*, Spring 2007; Kelley R, Where can $700 billion in waste be cut annually from the U.S. healthcare system? Thomson Reuters, October 2009.

15. World Health Organization. Core health indicators. http://www.who.int/countries/cri/en/. (Type title into Web site's search box.)

16. World Health Organization. Global atlas of the health workforce. http://www.who.int/globalatlas/default.asp.

17. World Health Organization: Core health indicators. http://www.who.int/countries/cri/en/ (Type title into Web site's search box.)

One

1. Findlay S. Military medicine. *U.S. News & World Report*, June 15, 1992, p. 72.

2. Wollstein J. Clinton's health-care plan for you: cradle-to-grave slavery. http://www.amatecon.com/etext/dosm/dosm-ch04.html.

3. Bauman RE. 70 years of federal government health care: a timely look at the U.S. Department of Veterans Affairs. Cato Policy Analysis No. 207. http://www.cato.org/pubs/pas/pa207es.html.

4. http://taxdayteaparty.com/2009/07/huge-announcing-the-nationwide-recess-rally/

5. Longman P. *The Return of Thrift: How the Collapse of the Middle Class Welfare State Will Reawaken Values in America*. New York: Free Press; 1996, chapter 10.

6. Jha AK, Perlin JB, Kizer KW, Dudley RA. Effect of the transformation of the veterans affairs health care system on the quality of care, *New England Journal of Medicine* 2003; 348:2218–2227. http://content.nejm.org/ (Type title into Web site's search box.)

7. Kerr E, Gerzoff R, Krein S, Selby J, Piette J, et al. A comparison of diabetes care quality in the veterans health care system and commercial managed care. *Annals of Internal Medicine* 2004; 141(4):272–281. http://www.annals.org/content/141/4/272.full

8. Asch SM, McGlynn EA, Hogan MM, Hayward RA, Shekelle P, Rubenstein L, Keesey J, Adams J, Kerr EA. Comparison of quality of

care for patients in the Veterans Health Administration and patients in a national sample. *Annals of Internal Medicine* 2004; 141(12): pp. 938–945.

9. Selim AJ, Kazis LE, Rogers W, Qian S, Rothendler JA, Lee A, Ren XS, Haffer SC, Mardon R, Miller D, Spiro A 3rd, Selim BJ, Fincke BG. Risk-adjusted mortality as an indicator of outcomes: comparison of the Medicare Advantage Program with the Veterans' Health Administration. Medical Care 2006; 44(4):359–365.

10. Ibid.

11. Oliver A, The Veterans Health Administration: an American success story? the *Milbank Quarterly*, vol. 85, no. 1, pp. 5–35 http://www.milbank.org/quarterly/8501feat.html (table 5)

12. Choi JC, Bakaeen FG, Huh J, Dao TK, LeMaire SA, Coselli JS, Chu D. Outcomes of coronary surgery at a Veterans Affairs hospital versus other hospitals. *J Surg Res*. 2009 Sep; 156(1):150–4.

13. Rehbein DK. A system worth saving: the condition of VA health care in America. 2009 Task Force Report. American Legion, Indianapolis, Indiana, 2009.

14. ACSI scores for U.S. federal government, American Customer Satisfaction Index I, December 15, 2006. http://www.theacsi.org/index.php?Itemid=160&id=164&option=com_content&task=view

15. Fact sheet: facts about the Department of Veterans Affairs, January 2009. http://www1.va.gov/opa/fact/vafacts.asp

16. Health IT strategic framework, attachment 2, III. The VA Electronic Health Record, VHA Office of Quality and Performance. http://www.hhs.gov/healthit/attachment_2/iii.html.

17. Leape LL, Berwick DM. Five years after *To Err Is Human*: what have we learned? *Journal of the American Medical Association* 2005; 293: 2384–2390.

18. Jha AK, Shlipak MG, et al. Racial differences in mortality among men hospitalized in the veterans affairs health care system, *Journal of the American Medical Association* 2001; 285:297–303.

19. Woolhandler S, Himmelstein DU. Competition in a publicly funded healthcare system. *BMJ* 2007; 335: 1126–1129

20. Healthcare program serving U.S. vets wins government innovation award: hi-tech Vista program one of two federal initiatives to win $100K grant. Press release, Ash Institute for Democratic Governance and Innovation at Harvard University's Kennedy School of Government. July 10, 2006. http://www.innovations.va.gov/innovations/docs/Harvard NewsRelease.pdf.

21. The health care system for veterans: an interim report. Congressional Budget Office, December 2007. http://www.cbo.gov/ftpdocs/88xx/doc8892/MainText.3.1.shtml, box 3.

22. Quality initiatives undertaken by the Veterans Health Administration, Congressional Budget Office. http://www.cbo.gov/ftpdocs/104xx/doc10453/08-13-VHA.pdf, Figure B-1

23. Department of Veterans Affairs, Congressional Submission, FY 2011 Funding and FY 2012 Advance Appropriations Request, Volume II, Medical Programs & Information Technology Programs, Executive Summary Charts, IB-2. www4.va.gov/budget/docs/summary/Fy2011_Volume_2-Medical_Programs_and_Information_Technology.pdf.

24. Trends in Health Care Costs and Spending, Kaiser Family Foundation, March 2009, Exhibit 1. www.kff.org/insurance/upload/7692_02.pdf.

25. Asch SM, et al. Who is at greatest risk for receiving poor-quality health care? *New England Journal of Medicine* 2006; 354:1147–1156. http://content.nejm.org/cgi/citmgr?gca=nejm;354/11/1147.

26. Ibid.

27. Oliver A, The Veterans Health Administration: an American success story? the *Milbank Quarterly*, vol. 85, no. 1

28. Jha AK, DesRoches CM, Campbell EG, Donelan K, Rao SR, Ferris TG, Shields A, Rosenbaum S, Blumenthal D. Use of electronic health records in U.S. hospitals, *New England Journal of Medicine* 2009; 360:1628–1638

29. Office of the Press Secretary, the White House. President Bush touts benefits of health care information technology. Department of Veterans Affairs Medical Center, Baltimore, MD, April 27, 2004.

Two

1. Russell R. *The Shadow of Blooming Grove: Warren G. Harding in His Times*. Norwalk, CT: Easton Press; 1988 (Reprint).

2. Daugherty HM. *The Inside Story of the Warren G. Harding Tragedy*. Whitefish, MT: Kessinger Publishing; 1960:179.

3. Quoted by Klein R. *Wounded Men, Broken Promises*. New York: Macmillan; 1981:41. *Only Yesterday*. New York: HarperCollins; 1931.

4. Klein, op. cit. p. 42.

5. Quoted by Klein, ibid., p. 42.

6. Department of Veterans Affairs, Office of Facilities Management. History of veterans healthcare.

7. Ibid.

8. The National Institutes of Health and The Veterans Administration. Advisory Committee on Human Radiation Experiments—Final Report, Chapter 1. http://www.eh.doe.gov/ohre/roadmap/achre/chap1_4.html; Lyon GM, Assistant Chief Medical Director for Research and

Education, presentation to the Committee on Veterans Medical Problems, National Research Council, December 8, 1952, Appendix II, Medical Research Programs of the Veterans Administration (ACHRE No. VA-052595-A).

9. Shortly before he died in 2001, an interviewer asked Ken Kesey how he first came to experiment with LSD. He answered: "I was connected to the VA hospital. Vic Lovell was working over there as a student of some kind, and when the drug experiment started, they set up a version of the VA hospital in Palo Alto. I went over and applied for a job, and a week or so later had a job. They put me on the same ward with the doctor that'd given me those early pills. He was not doing his experimentation anymore; he had quickly learned that this could be a real problem for the American government. One night, I came back in with my keys and went into his room, into his desk, and took out a lot of stuff. That was the source of most of our—all of our drugs—for a long time." See Digital Interviews Web site: http://www.digitalinterviews.com/digitalinterviews/views/kesey.shtml.

10. Quoted by Klein, ibid., p. 62.

Three

1. Chin T. Doctors pull plug on paperless system. *American Medical News*, Feb. 17, 2003.

2. Evans W. Associated Press, March 20, 1977.

3. Brown SH, et al. Vista-U.S. Department of Veterans Affairs national-scale HIS. *International Journal of Medical Informatics* 2003; 69:136–135.

4. Interview in Kenneth Dickie's home, Bethesda, MD, June 28, 2006.

5. Timson G. The history of the Hardhats. http://www.hardhats.org/history/hardhats.html.

6. Ibid.

7. Ibid.

8. Ibid.

9. Tomich N. Computers: new look at VA woes. *U.S. Medicine*, November 15, 1981.

10. Timson G. The history of the Hardhats. http://www.hardhats.org/history/hardhats.html.

11. Cited by Brown SH, et al. op. cit. p. 138.

12. Operating MUMP systems are integrated without hitch. *U.S. Medicine*, August 15, 1982, p. 1.

13. Timson G. The history of the Hardhats. http://www.hardhats .org/history/hardhats.html.

14. Tomich N. Congress urged to fund DHCP. *U.S. Medicine*, May 1987, p. 1.

Four

1. Interview by Spotswood S. Quality, access priorities in VA cancer care. *U.S. Medicine*, October, 2005. http://www.usmedicine.com/article .cfm?articleID=1167&issueID=80.

2. Remarks of Jonathan Perlin, Undersecretary for Health Affairs, Department of Veteran Affairs, to Ash Institute of the John F. Kennedy School of Government at Harvard University, July 10, 2006.

3. Spotswood S. VA flu vaccination plan prepares patients. *U.S. Medicine*, January 2006.

4. Management Brief, Health Services Research & Development Service, No. 6, December, 2002. http://www.research.va.gov/resources/ pubs/docs/hsr_brief_no6.pdf.

5. Khuri SF, et al. The Department of Veterans Affairs' NSQIP: the first national, validated, outcome-based, risk-adjusted, and peer-controlled program for the measurement and enhancement of the quality of surgical care. National VA Surgical Quality Improvement Program. *Annals of Surgery* 1998; 228(4):491–507.

6. Interviewed by Spangler D. VA electronic Rx records aid Katrina relief response. *U.S. Medicine*, November 2005. http://www.usmedicine .com/article.cfm?articleID=1202&issueID=81.

7. Oliver A. The Veterans Health Administration: an American success story? the *Milbank Quarterly*, vol. 85, no. 1. http://www.milbank .org/quarterly/8501feat.html.

Five

1. Editorial. More than veterans need. *St. Petersburg Times* (Florida), January 16, 1996, p. 10A.

2. Department of Veterans Affairs, Office of Inspector General. Audit of Veterans Health Administration resource allocation issues: physician staffing levels; 5R8-A19-113, September 29, 1995; Kilborn PT. Veterans expand hospital system in face of cuts. *New York Times*, January 14, 1996, sec. 1, p. 1, col. 3; National Desk.

3. Ibid.

4. Young GJ. Part three: the VHA transformation as viewed by Dr.

Kenneth W. Kizer, former Under Secretary for Health, U.S. Department of Veterans Affairs. http://www.businessofgovernment.org/pdfs/ Young_Report.pdf.

5. Office of the Assistant Deputy Under Secretary for Health. Vision for change: a plan to restructure the Veterans Health Administration. March 17, 1995. http://www4.va.gov/HEALTHPOLICYPLANNING/ VISION/2CHAP1.pdf.

6. Lichtenberg FR. Older Drugs, Shorter Lives? An Examination of the Health Effects of the Veterans Health Administration Formulary, Medical Progress Report, No. 2, October 2005. http://www.manhattan -institute.org/html/mpr_02.htm.

7. Blumenthal D, Herdman R, eds. VA Pharmacy Formulary Analysis Committee, Division of Health Care Services. *Description and Analysis of the VA National Formulary,* executive summary. Washington, DC: Institute of Medicine, National Academies Press; 2000.

8. Smith S. Recasting the lowly formulary. *Minnesota Medicine,* April 2006, vol. 89. www.minnesotamedicine.com/PastIssues/April2006/ QualityRoundsApril2006/tabid/2387/Default.aspx.

Six

1. CBO budget options, vol.1: health care. December 2008.

2. Corrigan J, et al., eds. *To Err Is Human: Building a Safer Health System.* Washington, DC: Institute of Medicine, the National Academies Press; 2000. http://darwin.nap.edu/books/0309068371/html/R1.html.

3. Centers for Disease Control and Prevention. Monitoring hospital-acquired infections to promote patient safety—United States, 1990–1999. Morbidity and Mortality Weekly Report 2000; 49:149–153.

4. Aspden P, et al. *Preventing Medication Errors.* Washington, DC: Institute of Medicine, the National Academies Press; 2007. http://darwin .nap.edu/books/0309101476/html.

5. Rand Corp. The First National Report Card on Quality of Health Care in America. http://www.rand.org/pubs/research_briefs/RB9053 -2/index1.html.

6. Office of the Medical Inspector, VHA. VA Patient Safety Event Registry: first nineteen months of reported cases summary and analysis, June 1997 through December 1998; Pear R. Report outlines medical errors in VA hospitals. *New York Times,* December 19, 1999, sec. 1, p. 1, col. 6.

7. Wiebe C. Patient safety concerns could spur bar code adoption. *Medscape Money & Medicine* 2002; 3(2).

8. Wood D. RN's visionary bar code innovation helps reduce medication errors. NurseZone.com, April 30, 2004. http://www.nursezone

.com/Nursing-News-Events/devices-and-technology/RN's-Visionary
-Bar-Code-Innovation-Helps-Reduce-Medication-Errors_24580.aspx.

9. Johnson CL, Carlson RA, Tucker CL, Willette C. Using BCMA
software to improve patient safety in Veterans Administration medical
centers. *Journal of Healthcare Information Management* 16(1). http://www
.himss.org/content/files/ambulatorydocs/BCMASoftwareToImprove-
PatientSafety.pdf.

10. Leape LL, Berwick DM. Five years after To Err Is Human: what
have we learned? *Journal of the American Medical Association* 2005; 293:
2384–2390.

Seven

1. Kleinke JD. Dot-gov: market failure and the creation of a national
health information technology system. *Health Affairs* 2005; 24(5):1246–
1262.

2. Casalino L. Markets and medicine: barriers to creating a "business
case for quality." *Perspectives in Biology and Medicine* 2002; 46(1):38–51.

3. Urbina I. In the treatment of diabetes, success often does not pay.
New York Times, January 11, 2006, p. 1. http://www.nytimes.com/
2006/01/11/nyregion/nyregionspecial5/11diabetes.html?pagewanted
=1&ei=5070&en=6c6db1d60e88d20b&ex=1148097600.

4. Snyderman R, Williams RW. The new prevention. *Modern Health-
care* 2003; 33:19.

5. Federal Trade Commission and the Department of Justice. Improving health care: a dose of competition. Report, July 2004, p. 24. http://
www.ftc.gov/reports/healthcare/040723healthcarerpt.pdf.

6. Leonhardt D. Making health care better, *New York Times Magazine*,
November 3, 2009, p. MM31.

7. World Wide Pursuing Perfection (WWPP). Pursuing perfection in
Whatcom County. http://www.wwpp.org:8080/wwppDiscuss/.

8. Homer J, et al. Models for collaboration: how system dynamics
helped a community organize cost-effective care for chronic illness. See
chart, p. 30. http://www.wwpp.org/static/gems/wwppDiscuss/sdp
.pdf#search=%22Models%20for%20 Collaboration%3A%20How%20Sys
tem %20Dynamics%20Helped%20%22.

9. Kolata G. Health plan that cuts costs raises doctors' ire. *New York
Times*, August 11, 2004. www.nytimes.com/pages/national/index.html.

10. Anderson GF, et al. Health care spending and use of information
technology in OECD countries. *Health Affairs* 2006; 25(3):819–831.

11. Brown SH, et al. *International Journal of Medical Informatics* 2003;

69:135–156, appendix B: Vista adopters outside of VA. http://www1.va.gov/cprsdemo/docs/Vista_Int_Jrnl_Article.pdf.

12. Rossi S. International expertise sought on e-health standards. *Computerworld: The Voice of IT Management.* (Australia). http://www.computerworld.com.au/index.php/id;358080262;fp;2;fpid;1.

13. Aldrich M. Safety First: *Technology, Labor, and Business in the Building of American Work Safety, 1870–1939.* Baltimore: Johns Hopkins University Press; 1997.

14. Bureau of Labor Statistics, National Compensation Survey Table 2. Medical care benefits: Access, participation, and take-up rates. March 2009 http://www.bls.gov/news.release/ebs2.t02.htm

15. Russell LB. Preventing chronic disease: an important investment, but don't count on cost savings. *Health Affairs*, January/February 2009; 28(1): 42–45.

16. Porter M, Olmsted TE. *Redefining Health Care: Creating Value-Based Competition on Results.* Cambridge, MA: Harvard Business School; 2006.

17. Sherman A, Greenstein R, Trisi D, Van de Water PN. Poverty rose, median income declined, and job-based health insurance continued to weaken in 2008. Center on Budget and Policy Priorities, September 10, 2009.

18. Payne JW. Your kind of doctor. *Washington Post*, January 31, 2006. http://www.washingtonpost.com/wp-dyn/content/article/2006/01/30/AR2006013001238.html.

19. Destiny Health, Opinion Research Corporation. Study reveals Americans resist doing healthcare homework; making more information available may not solve cost crisis. Press release. http://home.businesswire.com/portal/site/google/index.jsp?ndmViewId=news_view&newsId=20060814005734&newsLang=en.

20. Baker DW, Einstadter D, Thomas C, et al. The effect of publicly reporting hospital performance on market share and risk-adjusted mortality at high-mortality hospitals. *Medical Care* 2003; 41(6):729–740. http://www.ahrq.gov/research/oct03/ 1003RA3.htm.

Eight

1. Williams M. The doctor factor. *Washington Post*, December 31, 2003, p. A19.

2. Wennberg JE, Gittelsohn AM. Variations in medical care among small areas. *Science*, December 14, 1973, pp. 1102–1108.

3. Fitzhugh M. Wrestling with variation: an interview with Jack Wennberg. *Health Affairs* http://content.healthaffairs.org (Type title into Web site's search box.)

4. Fisher ES, Wennberg DE, Stukel TA, Gottlieb DJ, Lucas FL, Pinder EL. The implications of regional variations in Medicare spending, II: health outcomes and satisfaction with care. *Annals of Internal Medicine* 2003; 138:288–298.

5. Fisher ES, Wennberg DE, Stukel TA, Gottlieb DJ, Lucas FL, Pinder EL. The implications of regional variations in Medicare spending, I: the content, quality, and accessibility of care. *Annals of Internal Medicine* 2003; 138:273–287.

6. Gibbs N, Bower A. Q: What scares doctors? A: Being the patient. *Time*, May 1, 2006 (cover).

7. Roemer MI. Bed supply and hospital utilization: a natural experiment. *Hospitals* 1961; 35:36–42.

8. Abelson R. Heart procedure is off the charts in an Ohio city. *New York Times*, August 18, 2006, Business Desk. http://www.nytimes.com/2006/08/18/business/18stent.html?ex=1156996800&en=9a672c108ed8640c&ei=5070.

9. Gagnet K. Lourdes to pay $3.8M: hospital admits no fault in Patel-related matter. *Daily Advertiser* (Lafayette, La.), August 18, 2006.

10. Anderson-Cloud RL. Merging a divided system: the need to integrate care for individuals participating in both the Medicare and Medicaid Programs. *Age in Action*, Summer 1999. http://www.vcu.edu/vcoa/ageaction/agesu99.htm.

11. Ellwood P. Does managed care need to be replaced? Presentation to the Graduate School of Management, University of California, Irvine, October 2, 2001. http://www.medscape.com/viewarticle/408185.

12. Enthoven A. Review of *The Rise and Fall of HMOs: An American Health Care Revolution*, by Jan Gregoire Coombs. *CommonWealth*, Fall 2005. http://www.massinc.org/index.php?id=481&pub_id=1697&bypass=1.

13. Gruenberg EM. The failures of success. Paper presented as the Rema Lapouse lecture at the Annual Meeting of the American Public Health Association, Miami, Florida, October 19, 1976, reprinted in the *Milbank Memorial Fund Quarterly* 1977; 55(1):3–24. http://www.milbank.org/quarterly/830424gruenberg.pdf.

14. White K. The ecology of medical care: origins and implications for population-based healthcare. *Health Services Research* 1997; 32(1):11–21.

Nine

1. Remarks by Deputy Secretary W. Scott Gould, Connect Seminar '09, Washington, DC, June 30, 2009. http://www1.va.gov/opa/speeches/2009/09_0630_gould.asp; Memo from Executive Director, OI&T Field Operations & Development (005OP1) to VA OI&T Field

Operations and Developmental Staff. May 26, 2009 http://www.fred trotter.com/C3Moratorium.pdf.

2. Marshall F. Commentary: VA memo squashes VistA innovation, ModernHealthcare.com. (Type title in Web site's search box.)

3. O'Harrow Jr. R. The machinery behind health-care reform. *Washington Post*, May 16, 2009.

4. Zakaria S, Meyerson DA. How to fix health IT. *Washington Post* online, September 17, 2009. http://www.washingtonpost.com/wp-dyn/content/article/2009/09/17/ AR20090917 03734.html.

5. Blankenhorn D. VA now loves its VistA software. ZDNet Health care, October 15, 2009 http://healthcare.zdnet.com/?p=2836&tag =col1;post-2845.

6. Trotter F. http://www.fredtrotter.com/2009/04/28/ncvhs-testi mony-on-meaningful-use/.

Ten

1. Phone interview with Terry Nickel, wife of Gary Nickel. September 22, 2009, Moorhead, MN.

2. Remarks by Ambassador Michael W. Michalak. Agent Orange/Dioxin Joint Advisory Committee Results, The American Center, Hanoi, Vietnam, September 16, 2008. http://vietnam.usembassy.gov/amb speech091608.html.

3. Text of Clinton Statement on Veterans-Related Bills, Oct. 9, 1996. "The bill . . . authorizes the Department of Veterans Affairs to furnish comprehensive medical services to all veterans, expanding the array of services that it now provides. Eligibility reform has been a high priority of veterans for many years, and I am pleased that we finally could enact it." http://www.presidency.ucsb.edu/ws/index .php?pid=52074.

4. Physicians for a National Health Plan. Harvard researchers say 1.46 million working-age vets lacked health coverage last year, increasing their death rate. Press release, Nov. 10, 2009.

5. VetPop2007, Department of Veterans Affairs. http://www1.va .gov/VETDATA.

Eleven

1. Froomkim D. Mock the press, *Washington Post*, July 11, 2007. http://www.washingtonpost.com/wp-dyn/content/blog/2007/07/11/BL2007071101146 _pf.html.

2. Wilper AP, Woolhandler S, Lasser KE, McCormick D, Bor DH, Himmelstein DU. Health insurance and mortality in US adults. *Am J Public Health* 2009 0: AJPH.2008.157685.

3. Hadley J, Holahan J. Kaiser Commission on Medicaid and the uninsured, p. 4. http://www.kff.org/uninsured/upload/The-Cost-of-Care-for-the-Uninsured-What-Do-We-Spend-Who-Pays-and-What-Would-Full-Coverage-Add-to-Medical-Spending.pdf.

4. Asch SM et al. Who is at greatest risk for receiving poor-quality health care? *New England Journal of Medicine* 2006; 16:354(11): 1147–56.

5. Baker L, Atlas SW, Christopher CA. Expanded use of imaging technology and the challenge of measuring value. *Health Affairs* November/December 2008, 27(6): 1467-1478; Fazel R, Krumholz HM, Wang Y, et al. Exposure to low-dose ionizing radiation from medical imaging procedures. *New England Journal of Medicine* 2009; 361:849–857; Board on Radiation Effects Research, *Health Risks from Exposures to Low Levels of Ionizing Radiation: BEIR VII, Phase 2.* Washington, DC: National Academies Press; 2006.

6. Lauer MS. Elements of danger: the case of medical imaging. *New England Journal of Medicine* 2009; 361: 841–843.

7. Asch SM et al. Who is at greatest risk for receiving poor-quality health care? *New England Journal of Medicine* 2006; 16:354(11): 1147–56, table 3.

8. Frederick LA. *The Big Change: American Transforms Itself, 1900–1950.* New York: Harper; 1952: 202.

9. Fisher ES, Wennberg DE, Stukel TA, Gottlieb DJ, Lucas FL, Pinder EL. The implications of regional variations in Medicare spending, II: health outcomes and satisfaction with care. *Annals of Internal Medicine* 2003; 138:288–298.

10. Reinhardt U. Same surgery, different cost: insurance explained. Interview by Ari Shapiro, *Talk of the Nation,* National Public Radio, October 20, 2009. http://www.npr.org/templates/story/story.php?storyId=113971873.

11. Marmor TR. *The Politics of Medicare* (2nd edition). Hawthorne, New York: Aldine de Gruytor; 2000.

Epilogue

1. Mokdad AH, Marks JS, Stroup DF, Gerberding JL. Actual causes of death in the United States, 2000. *Journal of the American Medical Association* 2004; 291:1238–1245; Actual causes of death in the United States, 2000—correction. *Journal of the American Medical Association* 2005; 293:298.

2. Yasnoff WA. National health information infrastructure: key to the future of health care. U.S. Dept. of Health and Human Services; 2002.

3. Sherman SE, et al. Smokers' interest in quitting and services received: using practice information to plan quality improvement and policy for smoking cessation. *American Journal of Medical Quality* 2005; 20(1). http://ajm.sagepub.com/cgi/reprint/20/1/33.

4. Rules and Regulations, 38 CFR Part 17 RIN 2900–AM11. Elimination of copayment for smoking cessation counseling. *Federal Register,* vol. 70, no. 83.

5. For a fuller treatment of how medical privacy drives up the cost of private health insurance, see Longman P, Brownlee S. The genetic surprise. *Wilson Quarterly,* October 1, 2000.

Index

About the Author

Longman, a senior fellow at the New America Foundation, is the author of numerous articles and books on health care, demographics, and public policy. His most recent book (with Ray Boshara) is called *The Next Progressive Era: A Blueprint for Broad Prosperity* (2009). *The Empty Cradle* (2004) examines how the rapid yet uneven fall in birth rates around the globe is affecting the evolution of culture and politics. Mr. Longman is also the author of *Born to Pay: The New Politics of Aging in America* (1987) and *The Return of Thrift: How the Collapse of the Middle Class Welfare State Will Reawaken Values in America* (1996).

Mr. Longman's work has appeared in such publications as the *Atlantic, Financial Times, Foreign Affairs, Foreign Policy,* the *Harvard Business Review,* the *New Republic,* the *New York Times Magazine,* the *Wall Street Journal, Washington Monthly,* the *Washington Post,* and the *Wilson Quarterly.* He is a frequent public speaker, including addresses to the National War College, the Department of Health and Human Services, World Congress of Families, St. Galeen Forum, PopTech, Ford Hall Forum, and *Fortune* magazine's annual "Brainstorm" conference. He is also frequently interviewed by both foreign and domestic media, including National Public Radio, the

British Broadcasting Corporation, the Canadian Broadcasting Corporation, *Der Spiegel*, and many others. Formerly a senior writer and deputy assistant managing editor at *U.S. News & World Report*, he has won numerous awards for his business and financial writing, including UCLA's Gerald Loeb Award, and the top prize for investigative journalism from Investigative Reporters and Editors. He lives in Washington with his wife, Sandy, and son, Sam.

Other Books from PoliPointPress

*The Blue Pages: A Directory of Companies Rated by
Their Politics and Practices,* 2nd edition
Helps consumers match their buying decisions with their political values by list-
ing the political contributions and business practices of over 1,000 companies.
$12.95, PAPERBACK.

Sasha Abramsky, *Breadline USA: The Hidden Scandal
of American Hunger and How to Fix It*
Treats the increasing food insecurity crisis in America not only as a matter of
failed policies, but also as an issue of real human suffering. $23.95, CLOTH.

Rose Aguilar, *Red Highways: A Liberal's Journey into the Heartland*
Challenges red state stereotypes to reveal new strategies for progressives. $15.95,
PAPERBACK.

Dean Baker, *False Profits: Recovering from the Bubble Economy*
Recounts the causes of the economic meltdown and offers a progressive program
for rebuilding the economy and reforming the financial system and stimulus
programs. $15.95, PAPERBACK.

Dean Baker, *Plunder and Blunder: The Rise
and Fall of the Bubble Economy*
Chronicles the growth and collapse of the stock and housing bubbles and explains
how policy blunders and greed led to the catastrophic—but completely predictable—market meltdowns. $15.95, PAPERBACK.

Jeff Cohen, *Cable News Confidential:
My Misadventures in Corporate Media*
Offers a fast-paced romp through the three major cable news channels—Fox
CNN, and MSNBC—and delivers a serious message about their failure to cover
the most urgent issues of the day. $14.95, PAPERBACK.

Marjorie Cohn, *Cowboy Republic: Six Ways
the Bush Gang Has Defied the Law*
Shows how the executive branch under President Bush systematically defied the
law instead of enforcing it. $14.95, PAPERBACK.

Marjorie Cohn and Kathleen Gilberd, *Rules of Disengagement:
The Politics and Honor of Military Dissent*
Examines what U.S. military men and women have done—and what their families and others can do—to resist illegal wars, as well as military racism, sexual
harassment, and denial of proper medical care. $14.95, PAPERBACK.

Joe Conason, *The Raw Deal: How the Bush Republicans Plan to Destroy
Social Security and the Legacy of the New Deal*
Reveals the well-financed and determined effort to undo the Social Security Act
and other New Deal programs. $11.00, PAPERBACK.

Kevin Danaher, Shannon Biggs, and Jason Mark, *Building the Green Economy: Success Stories from the Grassroots*
Shows how community groups, families, and individual citizens have protected their food and water, cleaned up their neighborhoods, and strengthened their local economies. $16.00, PAPERBACK.

Kevin Danaher and Alisa Gravitz, *The Green Festival Reader: Fresh Ideas from Agents of Change*
Collects the best ideas and commentary from some of the most forward green thinkers of our time. $15.95, PAPERBACK.

Reese Erlich, *Dateline Havana: The Real Story of U.S. Policy and the Future of Cuba*
Explores Cuba's strained relationship with the United States, the island nation's evolving culture and politics, and prospects for U.S. Cuba policy with the departure of Fidel Castro. $22.95, HARDCOVER.

Reese Erlich, *The Iran Agenda: The Real Story of U.S. Policy and the Middle East Crisis*
Explores the turbulent recent history between the two countries and how it has led to a showdown over nuclear technology. $14.95, PAPERBACK.

Todd Farley, *Making the Grades: My Misadventures in the Standardized Testing Industry*
Exposes the folly of many large-scale educational assessments through an alternately edifying and hilarious firsthand account of life in the testing business. $16.95, PAPERBACK.

Steven Hill, *10 Steps to Repair American Democracy*
Identifies the key problems with American democracy, especially election practices, and proposes ten specific reforms to reinvigorate it. $11.00, PAPERBACK.

Jim Hunt, *They Said What? Astonishing Quotes on American Power, Democracy, and Dissent*
Covering everything from squashing domestic dissent to stymieing equal representation, these quotes remind progressives exactly what they're up against. $12.95, PAPERBACK.

Michael Huttner and Jason Salzman, *50 Ways You Can Help Obama Change America*
Describes actions citizens can take to clean up the mess from the last administration, enact Obama's core campaign promises, and move the country forward. $12.95, PAPERBACK.

Helene Jorgensen, *Sick and Tired: How America's Health Care System Fails Its Patients*
Recounts the author's struggle to receive proper treatment for Lyme disease and examines the inefficiencies and irrationalities that she discovered in America's health care system during that five-year odyssey. $16.95, PAPERBACK.

Markos Kounalakis and Peter Laufer, *Hope Is a Tattered Flag: Voices of Reason and Change for the Post-Bush Era*
Gathers together the most listened-to politicos and pundits, activists and thinkers, to answer the question: what happens after Bush leaves office? $29.95, HARDCOVER; $16.95 PAPERBACK.

Yvonne Latty, *In Conflict: Iraq War Veterans Speak Out on Duty, Loss, and the Fight to Stay Alive*
Features the unheard voices, extraordinary experiences, and personal photographs of a broad mix of Iraq War veterans, including Congressman Patrick Murphy, Tammy Duckworth, Kelly Daugherty, and Camilo Mejia. $24.00, HARDCOVER.

Phillip Longman, *Best Care Anywhere: Why VA Health Care Is Better Than Yours*
Shows how the turnaround at the long-maligned VA hospitals provides a blueprint for salvaging America's expensive but troubled health care system. $14.95, PAPERBACK.

Phillip Longman and Ray Boshara, *The Next Progressive Era*
Provides a blueprint for a re-empowered progressive movement and describes its implications for families, work, health, food, and savings. $22.95, HARDCOVER.

Marcia and Thomas Mitchell, *The Spy Who Tried to Stop a War: Katharine Gun and the Secret Plot to Sanction the Iraq Invasion*
Describes a covert operation to secure UN authorization for the Iraq war and the furor that erupted when a young British spy leaked it. $23.95, HARDCOVER.

Susan Mulcahy, ed., *Why I'm a Democrat*
Explores the values and passions that make a diverse group of Americans proud to be Democrats. $14.95, PAPERBACK.

David Neiwert, *The Eliminationists: How Hate Talk Radicalized the American Right*
Argues that the conservative movement's alliances with far-right extremists have not only pushed the movement's agenda to the right, but also have become a malignant influence increasingly reflected in political discourse. $16.95, PAPERBACK.

Christine Pelosi, *Campaign Boot Camp: Basic Training for Future Leaders*
Offers a seven-step guide for successful campaigns and causes at all levels of government. $15.95, PAPERBACK.

William Rivers Pitt, *House of Ill Repute: Reflections on War, Lies, and America's Ravaged Reputation*
Skewers the Bush Administration for its reckless invasions, warrantless wiretaps, lethally incompetent response to Hurricane Katrina, and other scandals and blunders. $16.00, PAPERBACK.

Sarah Posner, *God's Profits: Faith, Fraud, and the Republican Crusade for Values Voters*
Examines corrupt televangelists' ties to the Republican Party and unprecedented access to the Bush White House. $19.95, HARDCOVER.

Nomi Prins, *Jacked: How "Conservatives" Are Picking Your Pocket –Whether You Voted for Them or Not*
Describes how the "conservative" agenda has affected your wallet, skewed national priorities, and diminished America—but not the American spirit. $12.00, PAPERBACK.

Cliff Schecter, *The Real McCain: Why Conservatives Don't Trust Him—And Why Independents Shouldn't*
Explores the gap between the public persona of John McCain and the reality of this would-be president. $14.95, HARDCOVER.

Norman Solomon, *Made Love, Got War: Close Encounters with America's Warfare State*
Traces five decades of American militarism and the media's all-too-frequent failure to challenge it. $24.95, HARDCOVER.

John Sperling et al., *The Great Divide: Retro vs. Metro America*
Explains how and why our nation is so bitterly divided into what the authors call Retro and Metro America. $19.95, PAPERBACK.

Daniel Weintraub, *Party of One: Arnold Schwarzenegger and the Rise of the Independent Voter*
Explains how Schwarzenegger found favor with independent voters, whose support has been critical to his success, and suggests that his bipartisan approach represents the future of American politics. $19.95, HARDCOVER.

Curtis White, *The Barbaric Heart: Faith, Money, and the Crisis of Nature*
Argues that the solution to the present environmental crisis may come from unexpected quarters: the arts, religion, and the realm of the moral imagination. $16.95, PAPERBACK.

Curtis White, *The Spirit of Disobedience: Resisting the Charms of Fake Politics, Mindless Consumption, and the Culture of Total Work*
Debunks the notion that liberalism has no need for spirituality and describes a "middle way" through our red state/blue state political impasse. Includes three powerful interviews with John DeGraaf, James Howard Kunstler, and Michael Ableman. $24.00, HARDCOVER.

For more information, please visit www.p3books.com.

About This Book

This book is printed on Cascade Enviro100 Print paper. It contains 100 percent post-consumer fiber and is certified EcoLogo, Processed Chlorine Free, and FSC Recycled. For each ton used instead of virgin paper, we:

- Save the equivalent of 17 trees
- Reduce air emissions by 2,098 pounds
- Reduce solid waste by 1,081 pounds
- Reduce the water used by 10,196 gallons
- Reduce suspended particles in the water by 6.9 pounds.

This paper is manufactured using biogas energy, reducing natural gas consumption by 2,748 cubic feet per ton of paper produced.

The book's printer, Malloy Incorporated, works with paper mills that are environmentally responsible, that do not source fiber from endangered forests, and that are third-party certified. Malloy prints with soy and vegetable based inks, and over 98 percent of the solid material they discard is recycled. Their water emissions are entirely safe for disposal into their municipal sanitary sewer system, and they work with the Michigan Department of Environmental Quality to ensure that their air emissions meet all environmental standards.

The Michigan Department of Environmental Quality has recognized Malloy as a Great Printer for their compliance with environmental regulations, written environmental policy, pollution prevention efforts, and pledge to share best practices with other printers. Their county Department of Planning and Environment has designated them a Waste Knot Partner for their waste prevention and recycling programs.